T0188420

ANNALS *of* THE NEW YORK ACADEMY OF SCIENCES

EDITOR-IN-CHIEF
Douglas Braaten

ASSOCIATE EDITOR
Rebecca E. Cooney

PROJECT MANAGER
Steven E. Bohall

Artwork and design by Ash Ayman Shairzay

The New York Academy of Sciences
7 World Trade Center
250 Greenwich Street, 40th Floor
New York, NY 10007-2157

annals@nyas.org
www.nyas.org/annals

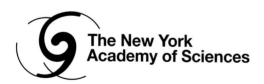

The New York
Academy of Sciences

Published by Blackwell Publishing
On behalf of the New York Academy of Sciences

Boston, Massachusetts
2012

ANNALS *of* THE NEW YORK ACADEMY OF SCIENCES

VOLUME
1275

ISSUE
Myasthenia Gravis and Related Disorders II
12th International Conference

ISSUE EDITORS
Gil I. Wolfe,[a] Matthew N. Meriggioli,[b] Emma Ciafaloni,[c] and Robert L. Ruff[d]

[a]University at Buffalo School of Medicine and Biomedical Sciences, [b]University of Illinois College of Medicine at Chicago, [c]University of Rochester Medical Center, and [d]Case Western Reserve University School of Medicine

TABLE OF CONTENTS

vii Introduction for *Myasthenia Gravis and Related Disorders*
Gil I. Wolfe, Matthew N. Meriggioli, Emma Ciafaloni, and Robert L. Ruff

Myasthenia gravis: treatment update and what lies ahead

1 IVIG and PLEX in the treatment of myasthenia gravis
Vera Bril, Carolina Barnett-Tapia, David Barth, and Hans D. Katzberg

7 Antigen-specific apheresis of autoantibodies in myasthenia gravis
Konstantinos Lazaridis, Paraskevi Zisimopoulou, George Lagoumintzis, Labrini Skriapa, Nikos Trakas, Panagiota Evangelakou, Ioannis Kanelopoulos, Eirini Grapsa, Kostas Poulas, and Socrates Tzartos

13 Further developments with antisense treatment for myasthenia gravis
Jon Sussman, Zohar Argov, Yitzhak Wirguin, Slobodan Apolski, Vedrana Milic-Rasic, and Hermona Soreq

17 Design of the Efficacy of Prednisone in the Treatment of Ocular Myasthenia (EPITOME) trial
Michael Benatar, Donald B. Sanders, Gil I. Wolfe, Michael P. McDermott, and Rabi Tawil

23 Phase II trial of methotrexate in myasthenia gravis
Mamatha Pasnoor, Jianghua He, Laura Herbelin, Mazen Dimachkie, Richard J. Barohn, and the Muscle Study Group

Congenital myasthenic syndromes

29 Identification of *DPAGT1* as a new gene in which mutations cause a congenital myasthenic syndrome
Katsiaryna Belaya, Sarah Finlayson, Judith Cossins, Wei Wei Liu, Susan Maxwell, Jacqueline Palace, and David Beeson

36 Synaptic basal lamina–associated congenital myasthenic syndromes
Ricardo A. Maselli, Juan Arredondo, Michael J. Ferns, and Robert L. Wollmann

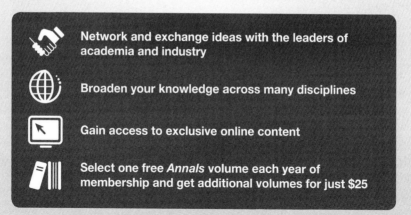

49   DOK7 congenital myasthenic syndrome
Jacqueline Palace

54   New horizons for congenital myasthenic syndromes
Andrew G. Engel, Xin-Ming Shen, Duygu Selcen, and Steven Sine

63   Synaptic dysfunction in congenital myasthenic syndromes
David Beeson

Lambert-Eaton myasthenic syndrome

70   SOX1 antibodies in Lambert–Eaton myasthenic syndrome and screening for small cell lung carcinoma
Alexander F. Lipka, Jan J.G.M. Verschuuren, and Maarten J. Titulaer

78   Treatment in Lambert–Eaton myasthenic syndrome
Paul Maddison

85   New calcium channel agonists as potential therapeutics in Lambert–Eaton myasthenic syndrome and other neuromuscular diseases
Tyler B. Tarr, Guillermo Valdomir, Mary Liang, Peter Wipf, and Stephen D. Meriney

Thymus, thymectomy, and the Myasthenia Gravis Thymectomy Trial

92   Thymus pathology observed in the MGTX trial
Alexander Marx, Frederik Pfister, Berthold Schalke, Wilfred Nix, and Philipp Ströbel

101   Biomarker development for myasthenia gravis
Henry J. Kaminski, Linda L. Kusner, Gil I. Wolfe, Inmaculada Aban, Greg Minisman, Robin Conwit, and Gary Cutter

107   Experimental myasthenia gravis in Aire-deficient mice: a link between Aire and regulatory T cells
Revital Aricha, Tali Feferman, Sonia Berrih-Aknin, Sara Fuchs, and Miriam C. Souroujon

Hot topics selected from submitted abstracts

114   Pathogenic IgG4 subclass autoantibodies in MuSK myasthenia gravis
Jaap J. Plomp, Maartje G. Huijbers, Silvère M. van der Maarel, and Jan J. Verschuuren

123   The search for new antigenic targets in myasthenia gravis
Judith Cossins, Katsiaryna Belaya, Katarzyna Zoltowska, Inga Koneczny, Susan Maxwell, Leslie Jacobson, Maria Isabel Leite, Patrick Waters, Angela Vincent, and David Beeson

129   Neuromuscular transmission failure in myasthenia gravis: decrement of safety factor and susceptibility of extraocular muscles
Alessandro Serra, Robert L. Ruff, and Richard John Leigh

Ann. N.Y. Acad. Sci. ISSN 0077-8923

Introduction for *Myasthenia Gravis and Related Disorders*

Myasthenia gravis (MG) is an acquired autoimmune syndrome caused by the failure of neuromuscular transmission, which results from the binding of autoantibodies to proteins involved in signaling at the neuromuscular junction (NMJ). Although the precise origin of the immune response in MG is not known, it remains one of the better characterized autoimmune disorders, and serves as a paradigm not only for understanding autoimmunity but also for the study of the NMJ and ion channels.

Earlier diagnosis and the availability of effective treatments have reduced the burden of high mortality and severe disability previously associated with myasthenia gravis. However, diagnosing the disease remains problematic and can be delayed because of its nonspecific and fluctuating symptoms. Furthermore, the management of MG is associated with considerable limitations. Treatment options in related myasthenic disorders are also inadequate. Present treatments for MG are either targeted toward symptoms or involve immunosuppressive therapies that have variable efficacy and that uniformly carry significant risk of infection or malignancy. Conventional treatments result in global, unfocused immunosuppression, rather than targeted inhibition of the autoreactive immune cells.

Myasthenia gravis and other disorders of the NMJ are relatively rare and are often neglected by national health authorities and the pharmaceutical industry. Held every five years, the International Conference on Myasthenia Gravis and Related Disorders attracts thought leaders in the field and provides a venue for researchers and clinicians to exchange ideas, establish collaborations, and continue to move the field forward. The international conferences also provide forums for younger investigators to communicate their recent findings.

The 12th International Conference on Myasthenia Gravis and Related Disorders was held on May 21–23, 2012 in New York City at the conference center at the New York Academy of Sciences. The meeting was cosponsored by the New York Academy of Sciences and the Myasthenia Gravis Foundation of America, with additional support provided by the NIH/NINDS/NCATS/ORD. Educational grants were received from Alexion Pharmaceuticals and BioMarin Pharmaceutical, Inc.; corporate sponsorships were received from CSL Behring, IBL International, KRONUS, Athena Diagnostics, and Terumo BCT. Nearly 300 scientists and clinicians from around the world attended the meeting.

The plenary sessions included 50 presentations. Over 100 abstracts were presented during two poster sessions. The keynote address by Marinos C. Dalakas summarized the evolution of biologics and other novel approaches in the treatment of MG and other immune-mediated neuromuscular disorders. Other highlights included latest developments pertaining to the structure of the NMJ; defects in regulatory T cells; the discovery of low-density lipoprotein receptor-related protein 4 as

doi: 10.1111/nyas.12013

an autoimmune target in MG; stem cell–mediated immunomodulation of lymphocytes derived from MG patients; recent basic and clinical findings in MuSK MG; the creation of patient registries; and updates on clinical trials, including the international thymectomy trial, acute management of MG exacerbations, methotrexate in MG, and preliminary investigations using complement inhibitors.

The four organizers of the conference would like to thank Brooke Grindlinger of the New York Academy of Sciences and Samuel Schulhof of the Myasthenia Gravis Foundation of America for their support of the three-day conference. Others who played integral roles include Melinda Miller and Melanie Koundourou, the New York Academy of Sciences, and Tor Holtan, the Myasthenia Gravis Foundation of America. Finally, we would like to acknowledge Douglas Braaten, editor-in-chief, *Annals of the New York Academy of Sciences,* for his help in assembling these proceedings.

GIL I. WOLFE

University at Buffalo School of Medicine and Biomedical Sciences, Buffalo, New York

MATTHEW N. MERIGGIOLI

University of Illinois College of Medicine at Chicago, Chicago, Illinois

EMMA CIAFALONI

University of Rochester Medical Center, Rochester, New York

ROBERT L. RUFF

Case Western Reserve University School of Medicine, Cleveland, Ohio

Ann. N.Y. Acad. Sci. ISSN 0077-8923

ANNALS OF THE NEW YORK ACADEMY OF SCIENCES

Issue: *Myasthenia Gravis and Related Disorders*

IVIG and PLEX in the treatment of myasthenia gravis

Vera Bril,[1] Carolina Barnett-Tapia,[1] David Barth,[2] and Hans D. Katzberg[1]

[1]Department of Medicine (Neurology), [2]Department of Pathology, University Health Network, University of Toronto, Toronto, Ontario, Canada

Address for correspondence: Vera Bril, Department of Medicine (Neurology), University Health Network, University of Toronto, 5EC-309, TGH, 200 Elizabeth Street, Toronto, ON, M5G 2C4, Canada. vera.bril@utoronto.ca

Intravenous immunoglobulin (IVIG) and plasma exchange (PLEX) are used to treat myasthenia gravis (MG) but with little trial evidence. While a class I study provided evidence for the efficacy of IVIG treatment, the empirical support for PLEX has been less convincing until recently. In a randomized controlled single-masked study of 84 MG patients with moderate to severe disease, IVIG and PLEX had comparable efficacy as demonstrated by reduction in the Quantitative Myasthenia Gravis Score (QMGS) for disease severity, percentage of responders, persistence of treatment effect, and tolerability, which were similar in both treatment arms. The change in QMGS was accompanied by improved disease-specific quality of life. The only factor predicting response to treatment was baseline severity. FcR polymorphisms did not predict response to IVIG therapy, but an inhibitory polymorphism was associated with baseline disease severity. These studies support the choice of either IVIG or PLEX as comparable treatments in adult patients with moderate to severe MG.

Keywords: myasthenia gravis; treatment; plasma exchange; plasmapheresis; intravenous immunoglobulin; comparison

Introduction

Myasthenia gravis (MG) is a prototype autoimmune disorder caused by anti-idiotype antibodies to acetylcholine receptors in 75% of patients, antimuscle specific kinase (anti-MuSK) antibodies in 5% of patients, and seronegative but immune treatment responsive in 20% of patients.[1–4] Both immunomodulation and immunosuppression are effective in treating patients with MG by removing anti-idiotype antibodies (plasma exchange, PLEX), resetting the immune system with intravenous immunoglobulin (IVIG), or suppressing the formation and action of abnormal antibodies (corticosteroids and other immunosuppressive drugs).[5–9] Despite the widespread use of these treatments in MG patients, few controlled trials have been done, and evidence for different interventions is lacking and needs to be developed.[10]

An adequately powered, class I study showed that IVIG, compared with placebo, is an effective treatment for MG,[9] and current guidelines support the use of IVIG in MG.[11,12] This is in contrast to the use of PLEX for MG. An older guideline stated that: "No adequate randomized controlled trials have been performed to determine whether PLEX improves the short-term or long-term outcome for MG."[5] More recently, an American Academy of Neurology (AAN) guideline update, published in 2011, suggests that the evidence is not robust for the use of PLEX in MG stating that: "There is insufficient evidence to support or refute the use of plasmapheresis in myasthenia gravis..." (Class III evidence, Level U).[8] A costing study suggests that IVIG is less expensive than PLEX in treating patients with MG.[13] Another unmasked study suggests that IVIG has fewer complications than PLEX.[14] Given these considerations, further evidence to support the use of PLEX in MG would be advantageous, particularly since some clinicians believe PLEX to be superior to IVIG, as suggested by a small uncontrolled series of patients.[15] The recent study by Barth *et al.*, published after the AAN guidelines, provides evidence in support for the use of PLEX in MG, showing outcomes comparable to those after IVIG treatment.[16]

doi: 10.1111/j.1749-6632.2012.06767.x

Ann. N.Y. Acad. Sci. 1275 (2012) 1–6 © 2012 New York Academy of Sciences.

IVIG and PLEX in MG

IVIG is an expensive treatment with multiple immune effects, such as a direct competition with anti-idiotype antibodies, anticomplement effects, or anti-Fc receptor effects.[17–19] IVIG is given intravenously and requires monitoring by nurses, often in specialized units. In MG, it is used mainly as a preoperative treatment or to treat patients with myasthenic exacerbation, myasthenic crises, or with refractory disease.[9,11,20] Although IVIG has been used in MG since the early 1980s, a controlled trial with placebo, randomization, and masked assessment was conducted only recently.[9,21,22]

PLEX is a method of removing abnormal antibody from plasma and has been used in MG since 1976.[23] This treatment requires specialized units, central venous access in some patients, and a long treatment interval of up to two weeks. Within this interval, five PLEX treatments are performed, with the removal of one plasma volume per treatment, to reduce antibody levels to low values. Consequently, it is an expensive therapy that is restricted to specialized units. PLEX is used, similarly to IVIG, mainly for preoperative preparation of patients, and the treatment of patients with myasthenic crises and refractory MG.[24]

Clinical experience shows that both IVIG and PLEX lead to short-term improvement in MG patients. Early trial evidence on these treatments was based on small numbers of patients and open treatment without placebo arms.[5,8,15] PLEX became the standard immunomodulation in MG patients before the introduction of IVIG and was widely used despite the lack of high-level evidence of its usefulness, but rather on the basis of its reported efficacy for patients in crisis.[15,25] Even after the introduction of IVIG, many experts still consider PLEX the best option and do not consider IVIG for the treatment of severely ill patients or in preoperative preparation. The Zinman study was a placebo-controlled, masked evaluator, randomized, and adequately powered study that confirmed the benefits of IVIG in moderate to severe MG.[9] In contrast, PLEX for the treatment of MG has still not been evaluated in a similar fashion using a sham-exchange controlled arm and masked evaluation; the studies on PLEX to date have been open studies or retrospective reports excepting the recent report by Barth.[16]

IVIG versus PLEX: efficacy

Studies comparing IVIG to PLEX showed variable results with some reports favoring PLEX treatment, and others showing comparable outcomes with both treatments.[14,25] However, no masked assessor studies had been done, and the course of PLEX treatment was less than standard in some centers. A second study was undertaken in our center to compare the efficacy of IVIG and PLEX in reducing disease severity in MG patients requiring a change in therapy due to worsening disease.[16] This study was a masked evaluator (single-blind) study because it was considered to not fit clinical equipoise to include sham exchange as a comparator for PLEX, or placebo as a comparator for IVIG, given the results of the prior study establishing the benefits of IVIG. An *a priori*, predefined, clinically significant difference in outcomes between the two treatment arms of >3.5 units on the mean Quantitative Myasthenia Gravis Score (QMGS) was required to find one treatment better than the other. This degree of change in the QMGS had been determined previously to be clinically significant by experts in the field and is approximately a 10% change in the scale ranging from 0 to 39 points.[26] The study enrolled and randomized 84 patients with moderate to severe MG to receive IVIG 2 g/kg over two days or PLEX, one plasma volume per treatment repeated five times within about 10 days. The patients were assessed at day 14 after treatment was completed in contrast to other comparison studies that assessed MG status at different time points after treatment or evaluated hospital length of stay or comorbid diseases.[13,14,25] The reduction in disease severity or change in QMGS was: 3.2 ± 4.1 (CI: 2–4.5) for IVIG and 4.7 ± 4.9 (CI: 3.2–6.2) for PLEX, $P = 0.13$, and thus not clinically significantly different between the two patient arms. The postintervention status showed that 69% of patients responded to IVIG and 65% to PLEX, a difference that was not significant. This study provides class I evidence that IVIG and PLEX are comparable in treatment effects when given to patients with moderate to severe MG.[16]

Some other important observations from this study are that none of the patients required additional treatment up to day 14, in either treatment arm. The treatment effect was maintained until day 28 in both arms, as shown in Figure 1. The drop out rate was the same in both arms, and the same

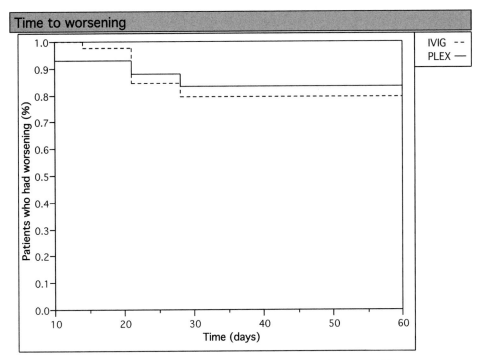

Figure 1. Kaplan–Meier curve for persistence of treatment effect after treatment with IVIG or PLEX.

number of patients needed additional treatment in each arm. The dropout rate between days 14 and 60 was 10 patients on IVIG (8 with worsening disease) and 9 patients on PLEX (7 with worsening disease), χ^2, $P = 0.79$. So, even when considering the overall clinical course, differences favoring one treatment over another were not discovered in this cohort of MG patients.

IVIG versus PLEX: safety

Important concerns about PLEX are the vascular access and safety compared to IVIG, as some reports indicate that IVIG is associated with fewer serious adverse events.[13] In the Barth study, 83% of patients completed all PLEX treatment via peripheral venous access and no premedication was used for any of the treatments.[27] Ten percent of patients had all treatments by central venous access and 7% changed from peripheral to central access. Ninety percent of patients completed their treatment as outpatients, and the 10% treated as inpatients had been admitted as impending myasthenic crises rather than for purposes of receiving PLEX. Fifty-five percent of the patients did not have any adverse reactions, but those that occurred were primarily grade I or II, that

is, mostly mild and easily treated without stopping PLEX.[28] The most serious adverse events occurred in the PLEX group. One 69-year-old male participant had prior coronary artery disease with myocardial infarction, bypass graft, percutaneous coronary angioplasty, and stenting. He had neck pain and was found to have had a myocardial infarction. This event was considered probably related to the treatment. The other was an 83-year-old female with preexisting diabetes, hypertension, congestive heart failure (controlled), and hypercholesterolemia. She developed pneumonia and exacerbation of congestive heart failure within one week after completing all PLEX sessions. This event was considered to be unrelated to the treatment.

The most common comorbid disease was hypertension (35.7%), followed by diabetes mellitus (11.9%). Comorbid disorders did not predict adverse events during treatment.

IVIG versus PLEX: quality of life

The primary outcome measure used in this study was the change in the QMGS with a decrease indicating reduced MG severity.[26] However, severity in MG also negatively affects various psychological, social, and functional aspects of daily living that are not captured directly by the QMGS but are reflected in disease specific quality of life (Myasthenia Gravis-Quality of Life, MG-QOL) scales.[29] The impact of treatment on change in MG-QOL might influence the choice of IVIG or PLEX. This question was examined in patients from the Barth study, which found that changes in the MG-QOL-60 and MG-QOL-15 were similar in both treatments, with a decrease (meaning improved quality of life) at day 14 continuing to day 60. The MG-QOL scores were lower for responders than nonresponders (defined by the change in the QMGS score) and also corresponded to the postintervention status (lower in those who improved compared to those who stayed the same or worsened).[30] The comparable benefits in terms of quality of live improvement eliminates quality of life as a factor to consider when choosing between IVIG and PLEX in a given patient.

Predictors of response to immunomodulation

The QMGS, the primary efficacy parameter in this study, has been used in several MG studies after the recommendations of the MG Foundation of America (MGFA).[9,16,26,31,32] This is a quantitative measure of elements of the clinical examination based on expert opinion. We have observed that the QMGS correlates well with the MGFA classification of disease categories ($r^2 = 0.54$, $P < 0.0001$ with a pooled 95% CI of I: 5.2–9.9, II: 10.8–12.2, III: 16.0–17.7, IV: 14.8–27.1, and V: 23.8–36.1) but is not influenced by age, gender, disease duration, history of thymoma, or current medications. Furthermore, we have observed a moderate correlation of QMGS with MG-QOL-15 ($r^2 = 0.41$, $P = 0.0007$) and a good correlation with another biomarker of disease, the single fiber jitter ($r^2 = 0.40$, $P < 0.0001$).[33,34] Correlations with the percent of abnormal pairs and the percent of blocking pairs were also observed, but none between the QMGS and acetylcholine receptor antibody (AChRAb) titers, although the QMGS was higher in those positive for AChRAb compared to seronegative patients (14.2 ± 4.5 compared to 12.0 ± 3.7, $P = 0.008$).[33] In our experience, the QMGS for disease severity is a valid biomarker of the severity of MG, as indicated by the MGFA scale, MG-QOL-15, electrophysiological markers, and serological status. Our observations support the use of the QMGS as an efficacy parameter in clinical trials of MG, and newer tools should have performance characteristics of equal quality to the QMGS to be used in future trials.[33]

It is important to note that not all patients respond to either IVIG or PLEX, so that any factors that predict who would respond would also be useful to help select a therapy in the clinic. In a comprehensive analysis of predictors of response to immunomodulation, we evaluated patients from the previous MG studies (IVIG compared to placebo and IVIG compared to PLEX)[9,16] with regard to factors such as age, gender, medications, history of thymoma, baseline disease severity, and history of thymectomy that might predict response to treatment (Table 1). We found that in bivariate analyses, baseline QMGS, single fiber electromyography parameters (jitter, % abnormal pairs, % blocking pairs), and AChRab positivity predicted responder status. However, in multivariable regression analyses, only baseline disease severity predicted who would respond to therapy, with an odds ratios of 13.0 (95% CI: 1.02–381.5) for QMGS 11–16 and 15.3 (95% CI: 1.34–414.3) for QMGS >16 when using QMGS <11 as a reference.[35] Although regression to the mean and defining "responders" at the lower levels of disease severity (currently being further investigated) may have played a minor role in this finding, there does seem to be a more robust effect of treatment with higher baseline QMGS; AChRab positivity and single fiber electromyography (SFEMG) likely simply reflect more advanced disease severity. It is important to note that 25% of AChRab-negative patients responded to therapy, which indicated that patients who are seronegative may still respond robustly to immunomodulation and should not be denied access to treatment. This study had only small numbers of MuSK-positive patients and equal numbers responded or failed to respond to therapy in this cohort. As such, it is difficult to make any comments on whether this subgroup of patients responds favorably to immunomodulation. We also analyzed certain polymorphisms in the Fc receptor (FcR) to determine if any predicted those who would respond to treatment with IVIG. None of the FcR polymorphisms studied predicted response to IVIG, but patients with the FCγR2B-232I/I polymorphism had higher disease severity scores measured by the QMGS.[36] This observation suggests a double-negative immune effect, as this receptor has an inhibitory role and this polymorphism

Table 1. Baseline variables predictive of response to immunomodulatory treatment in patients with MG using bivariate analysis

Parameter	Nonresponder ($n = 46$)	Responder ($n = 57$)	P value
Demographics:			
Gender (F %)	61	49	0.22
Age	55.1	59.9	0.12
Disease duration (months)	72.6	57.1	0.32
Baseline clinical status:			
QMGS (baseline)	12.4	14.9	0.003
Previous thymectomy	32.6	38.2	0.84
Thymus status:			
Thymoma (%)	25	25.4	0.55
Previous treatments:			
Previous IGIV (%)	13.6	14.5	0.90
Previous PLEX (%)	18.2	10.9	0.30
Current treatments:			
Currently on pyridostigmine (%)	50.0	61.1	0.12
Currently on prednisone (%)	45.5	36.4	0.36
Currently on azathioprine (%)	29.6	14.6	0.07
Currently on mycophenylate mofetil (%)	11.4	1.8	0.05
Electrophysiology:			
Repetitive nerve stimulation:			
Baseline decrement (%)	12.0	18.3	0.10
Immediately postexercise (%)	13.7	16.7	0.12
Decrement one minute after exercise (%)	13.4	19.2	0.13
Single fiber EMG:			
Jitter (μs)	86.6	122.5	0.0005
Abnormal pairs (%)	59.3	76.9	0.002
Blocking pairs (%)	9.6	18.9	0.002
Antibody status:			
AchRAb$^+$ (%)	55.0	84.9	0.001
AchRAb titres (μmol/L)	166.2	209.1	0.18
MuSK$^+$ (%)	7.5	5.6	0.72
Seronegative patients (AChRAb–MuSK$^-$) (%)	37.5	7.7	0.005

AChRAb, acetylcholine receptor antibody; MuSK, muscle specific kinase; RNS, repetitive nerve stimulation.

confers higher affinity. However, these findings require confirmation in a larger patient cohort.

Conclusions

In summary, our studies have confirmed that IVIG is an effective treatment for MG patients with worsening weakness and that IVIG and PLEX have comparable outcomes in treating MG patients with moderate to severe weakness that requires a change in therapy. Both treatments reduce the severity of clinical disease, improve quality of life, improve biomarkers of disease, and are well tolerated. Neither treatment requires hospitalization. Our study suggests that either treatment can be selected depending on availability of resources and individual patients' characteristics that would preclude the use of a given treatment.

Conflicts of interest

The authors declare no conflicts of interest.

References

1. Vincent, A., J. McConville, M.E. Farrugia, *et al.* 2003. Antibodies in myasthenia gravis and related disorders. *Ann. N. Y. Acad. Sci.* **998:** 324–335.
2. Vincent, A., J. Palace & D. Hilton-Jones. 2001. Myasthenia gravis. *Lancet* **357:** 2122–2128.
3. Vincent, A. & M.I. Leite. 2005. Neuromuscular junction autoimmune disease: muscle specific kinase antibodies and treatments for myasthenia gravis. *Curr. Opin. Neurol.* **18:** 519–525.
4. Hohlfeld, R. & H. Wekerle. 1999. The Immunopathogenesis of myasthenia gravis. In *Myasthenia Gravis and Myasthenic Disorders.* A.G. Engel, Ed.: 87–104. Oxford University Press. New York.
5. Gajdos, P., S. Chevret & K. Toyka. 2002. Plasma exchange for myasthenia gravis. *Cochrane. Database Syst. Rev.* CD002275.
6. Lisak, R.P. 1984. Plasma exchange in neurologic diseases. *Arch. Neurol.* **41:** 654–657.
7. Keesey, J.C. 2004. Clinical evaluation and management of myasthenia gravis. *Muscle Nerve* **29:** 484–505.
8. Cortese, I., V. Chaudhry, Y.T. So, *et al.* 2011. Evidence-based guideline update: plasmapheresis in neurologic disorders: report of the Therapeutics and Technology Assessment Subcommittee of the American Academy of Neurology. *Neurology* **76:** 294–300.
9. Zinman, L., E. Ng & V. Bril. 2007. IV immunoglobulin in patients with myasthenia gravis: a randomized controlled trial. *Neurology* **68:** 837–841.
10. Miller, R.G., R.J. Barohn & R. Dubinsky. 2010. Expanding the evidence base for therapeutics in myasthenia gravis. *Ann. Neurol.* **68:** 776–777.
11. Gajdos, P., S. Chevret & K. Toyka. 2008. Intravenous immunoglobulin for myasthenia gravis. *Cochrane. Database Syst. Rev.* CD002277.
12. Patwa, H.S., V. Chaudhry, H. Katzberg, *et al.* 2012. Evidence-based guideline: intravenous immunoglobulin in the treatment of neuromuscular disorders: report of the Therapeutics and Technology Assessment Subcommittee of the American Academy of Neurology. *Neurology* **78:** 1009–1015.
13. Mandawat, A., H.J. Kaminski, G. Cutter, *et al.* 2010. Comparative analysis of therapeutic options used for myasthenia gravis. *Ann. Neurol.* **68:** 797–805.
14. Gajdos, P., S. Chevret, B. Clair, *et al.* 1997. Clinical trial of plasma exchange and high-dose intravenous immunoglobulin in myasthenia gravis. Myasthenia Gravis Clinical Study Group. *Ann. Neurol.* **41:** 789–796.
15. Stricker, R.B., B.J. Kwiatkowska, J.A. Habis & D.D. Kiprov. 1993. Myasthenic crisis. Response to plasmapheresis following failure of intravenous gamma-globulin. *Arch. Neurol.* **50:** 837–840.
16. Barth, D., M. Nabavi Nouri, E. Ng, *et al.* 2011. Comparison of IVIg and PLEX in patients with myasthenia gravis. *Neurology* **76:** 2017–2023.
17. Ephrem, A., S. Chamat, C. Miquel, *et al.* 2008. Expansion of CD4+CD25+ regulatory T cells by intravenous immunoglobulin: a critical factor in controlling experimental autoimmune encephalomyelitis. *Blood* **111:** 715–722.
18. Soueidan, S.A. & M.C. Dalakas. 1993. Treatment of autoimmune neuromuscular diseases with high-dose intravenous immune globulin. *Pediatr. Res.* **33:** S95–S100.
19. Anthony, R.M., F. Wermeling, M.C. Karlsson & J.V. Ravetch. 2008. Identification of a receptor required for the anti-inflammatory activity of IVIG. *Proc. Natl. Acad. Sci. USA* **105:** 19571–19578.
20. Jensen, P. & V. Bril. 2008. A comparison of the effectiveness of intravenous immunoglobulin and plasma exchange as preoperative therapy of myasthenia gravis. *J. Clin. Neuromuscul. Dis.* **9:** 352–355.
21. Dau, P.C. 1983. Immune globulin intravenous replacement after plasma exchange. *J. Clin. Apher.* **1:** 104–108.
22. Fateh-Moghadam, A., M. Wick, U. Besinger & R.G. Geursen. 1984. High-dose intravenous gammaglobulin for myasthenia gravis. *Lancet* **1:** 848–849.
23. Pinching, A.J. & D.K. Peters. 1976. Remission of myasthenia gravis following plasma-exchange. *Lancet* **2:** 1373–1376.
24. Skeie, G.O., S. Apostolski, A. Evoli, *et al.* 2010. Guidelines for treatment of autoimmune neuromuscular transmission disorders. *Eur. J. Neurol.* **17:** 893–902.
25. Qureshi, A.I., M.A. Choudhry, M.S. Akbar, *et al.* 1999. Plasma exchange versus intravenous immunoglobulin treatment in myasthenic crisis. *Neurology* **52:** 629–632.
26. Tindall, R.S., J.T. Phillips, J.A. Rollins, *et al.* 1993. A clinical therapeutic trial of cyclosporine in myasthenia gravis. *Ann. N. Y. Acad. Sci.* **681:** 539–551.
27. Ebadi, H., D. Barth & V. Bril. In Press. Safety of plasma exchange therapy in patients with myasthenia gravis. *Muscle Nerve.*
28. Norda, R., B.G. Stegmayr, Swedish Apheresis Group. 2003. Therapeutic apheresis in Sweden: update of epidemiology and adverse events. *Transfus. Apher. Sci.* **29:** 159–166.
29. Mullins, L.L., M.Y. Carpentier, R.H. Paul & D.B. Sanders. 2008. Disease-specific measure of quality of life for myasthenia gravis. *Muscle Nerve* **38:** 947–956.
30. Barnett, C., G. Wilson, D. Barth, *et al.* In Press. Changes in MG-QOL with IVIG or plasmapheresis in patients with myasthenia gravis. *J. Neurol. Neurosurg. Psychiatry.*
31. Jaretzki, A. 3rd, R.J. Barohn, R.M. Ernstoff, *et al.* 2000. Myasthenia gravis: recommendations for clinical research standards. Task Force of the Medical Scientific Advisory Board of the Myasthenia Gravis Foundation of America. *Ann. Thorac. Surg.* **70:** 327–334.
32. Sanders, D.B., I.K. Hart, R. Mantegazza, *et al.* 2008. An international, phase III, randomized trial of mycophenolate mofetil in myasthenia gravis. *Neurology* **71:** 400–406.
33. Barnett, C., H. Katzberg, M. Nabavi & V. Bril. 2012. The quantitative myasthenia gravis score: comparison with clinical, electrophysiological & laboratory markers. *J. Clin. Neuromuscul. Dis.* **13:** 201–205.
34. Zinman, L., D. Baryshnik & V. Bril. 2008. Surrogate therapeutic outcome measures in patients with myasthenia gravis. *Muscle Nerve* **37:** 172–176.
35. Katzberg, H.D., C. Barnett & V. Bril. 2012. Predictors of response to immunomodulation in patients with myasthenia gravis. *Muscle Nerve* **45:** 648–652.
36. Barnett, C., Y. Grinberg, M. Ghani, *et al.* 2012. Fcgamma receptor polymorphisms do not predict response to intravenous immunoglobulin in myasthenia gravis. *J. Clin. Neuromuscular. Dis.* **14:** 1–6.

Ann. N.Y. Acad. Sci. ISSN 0077-8923

ANNALS OF THE NEW YORK ACADEMY OF SCIENCES

Issue: *Myasthenia Gravis and Related Disorders*

Antigen-specific apheresis of autoantibodies in myasthenia gravis

Konstantinos Lazaridis,[1] Paraskevi Zisimopoulou,[1] George Lagoumintzis,[1] Labrini Skriapa,[1,2] Nikos Trakas,[1] Panagiota Evangelakou,[1,2] Ioannis Kanelopoulos,[1,2] Eirini Grapsa,[3] Kostas Poulas,[2] and Socrates Tzartos[1,2]

[1]Hellenic Pasteur Institute, Athens, Greece. [2]University of Patras, Patras, Greece. [3]Department of Nephrology, Aretaieion University Hospital, Athens, Greece

Address for correspondence: Socrates J. Tzartos, Hellenic Pasteur Institute, 127 Vas. Sofias Ave., Athens, 11521, Greece. tzartos@mail.pasteur.gr

Myasthenia gravis (MG) is an autoimmune disorder affecting the neuromuscular junction, usually caused by autoantibodies against the acetylcholine receptor (AChR) or the muscle-specific kinase (MuSK). Our aim is the development of a therapy based on the selective extracorporeal elimination of anti-AChR or anti-MuSK antibodies. To this end, the extracellular domains of the AChR subunits and MuSK have been expressed in yeast to be used as adsorbents, after optimization, and to obtain large quantities of proteins with near-native structure. We have characterized these proteins with respect to their use as specific immunoadsorbents for MG autoantibodies, and have begun large-scale experiments in order to verify the feasibility of application of the method for therapy. Furthermore, we have initiated animal studies to test possible toxicity and safety issues of the adsorbents or the procedure itself. The successful completion of the scale-up and safety tests will allow the initiation of clinical trials.

Keywords: myasthenia gravis; antigen-specific immunoadsorption; acetylcholine receptor; muscle-specific kinase; extracellular domain; therapy

Introduction

Myasthenia gravis (MG) is a prototype antibody-mediated autoimmune disease targeting the neuromuscular junction (NMJ) of skeletal muscles. This causes impairment of signal transduction from the nerve terminal, which in turn leads to muscle weakness and fatigability. When the respiratory muscles are affected it results in reduced ventilation capacity, which in severe cases can progress to a myasthenic crisis, a potentially life-threatening condition.

In the majority of patients ($\sim$85%) the antigen targeted is the muscle nicotinic acetylcholine receptor (AChR).[1] The AChR is an ion channel composed of five subunits, with the stoichiometry $(\alpha 1)_2 \beta 1 \gamma \delta$ for fetal or denervated muscles and $(\alpha 1)_2 \beta 1 \varepsilon \delta$ for adult muscles.[2] Most of the antigenic epitopes are located on the extracellular domains of the AChR subunits (ECDs), while more

than half of the autoantibodies are directed against the so-called main immunogenic region (MIR), a group of overlapping epitopes located on the ECD of the $\alpha 1$ subunit, whose central core lies between amino acids 67 and 76, although other segments contribute as well.[3,4] The structure of the MIR promotes binding of conformation-dependent MG autoantibodies, AChR conformation maturation, and agonist sensitivity.[5] Although antibodies against intracellular or transmembrane epitopes have been found, they are probably not clinically important since these epitopes are inaccessible in undamaged muscle membranes. The pathogenicity of the anti-AChR antibodies has been shown by their ability to cause experimental MG when injected into rats, and by the clinical improvement of patients after plasmapheresis.[6–8]

In another $\sim$6% of MG patients, the autoantibodies are directed against the muscle-specific

doi: 10.1111/j.1749-6632.2012.06788.x

kinase (MuSK), a muscle membrane protein, which mediates AChR clustering at the NMJ.[9] The remaining ~10% of diagnosed MG patients do not have detectable anti-AChR or anti-MuSK antibodies and are accordingly referred to as seronegative. It is thought that they have autoantibodies directed against other proteins of the NMJ, or low levels of antibodies against the known targets, which cannot be detected. Indeed, recently it was shown that low affinity anti-AChR antibodies can be found in some previously seronegative patients using more sensitive detection assays, such as a cell-based assay.[10] In the case of MuSK-MG our team has developed a highly sensitive test in the form of a two-step radioimmuno-precipitation assay, which can detect very low consentrations of anti-MuSK antibodies.[11] On the other hand, a fraction of the remaining patients were shown by several groups, including our team, to have antibodies against a novel autoantigen, the low-density lipoprotein receptor-related protein 4 (LRP4).[12–14] LRP4 is involved together with MuSK in the AChR-clustering signaling pathway.

The most common treatment strategies for MG currently include the use of cholinesterase inhibitors, immunosuppressives, thymectomy, intravenous immunoglobulin (IVIG), and plasmaphereses.[15] These are largely nonspecific and thus may be accompanied by a variety of side effects.

Plasmapheresis is commonly used in MG patients who are refractory to other therapies or when an immediate effect is needed (myasthenic crisis, preoperative treatment) as it provides a fast, albeit temporary, improvement of muscle weakness.[16] It involves the removal of plasma from the patients, thus reducing the autoantibodies from the patients' circulation. This, however, results in the removal of all plasma components, including plasma proteins and protective antibodies. Moreover, the plasma albumin needs to be replaced, increasing the risk of allergic reactions and transfusion-related infections.

A procedure related to plasmapheresis is immunoadsorption—the extracorporeal removal of immunoglobulins from the patient's blood. This is achieved by passage of the plasma through a suitable matrix to bind the immunoglobulins and then return the plasma to the patient. Although this does not remove most plasma components and alleviates the need for replacements, it still results in the removal of all immunoglobulins indiscriminately, including any protective antibodies. Commonly

used matrices for this approach include antihuman IgG or protein A immobilized onto sepharose beads.[17,18]

An attractive alternative would be the selective removal of only the autoantibodies (antigen-specific immunoadsorption). This could be achieved by use of a suitable matrix, such as immobilized autoantigens (Fig. 1). To this end, the ECDs of the autoantigens are preferable since they are easier to express than the full length transmembrane molecules.[19]

We have described the expression of the ECDs of the AChR subunits and MuSK in the yeast *P. pastoris* as secreted soluble proteins with near-native structure.[20,21] Furthermore, it was shown that immobilized onto sepharose beads they can bind autoantibodies from patients' sera,[11,22,23] and that depletion of the sera from the autoantibodies was sufficient to ablate their antigen modulating activity in cultures of TE761 cells.[24]

In this report we present data on more extensive characterization of the adsorbents, such as modifications for improved expression, capacity for autoantibodies, and ability to be regenerated by elution of bound antibodies. Furthermore, we examined the upscaling of the procedure using large volumes of plasma and high flow rates comparable to those used in clinical practice. Finally, we have addressed a series of safety aspects, including adsorbent toxicity and the possibility of adverse reactions due to the procedure in experimental animals. Results presented herein strongly support the feasibility of the development of this specific apheresis method for the treatment of MG patients.

AChR immmunoadsorbents

Expression of ECD adsorbents in yeast
Initial attempts to express the ECDs of the AChR in yeast showed that they had a near-native structure, but with the exception of the β1-ECD, they were produced at relatively low levels.[20,21] On the other hand, *Escherichia coli* expressed ECDs had a much higher yield, but their reduced efficiency made their clinical use problematic.[25] We, therefore, proceeded with a series of mutations in one of the proteins, the γ-ECD, aiming at making it more hydrophilic.[26] We found that the most striking effect was achieved when the so-called cys-loop of the γ-ECD was exchanged with that of the acetylcholine binding protein (AChBP) from the snail *Lymnaea stagnalis*, a soluble homolog of the AChRs. This mutation led to

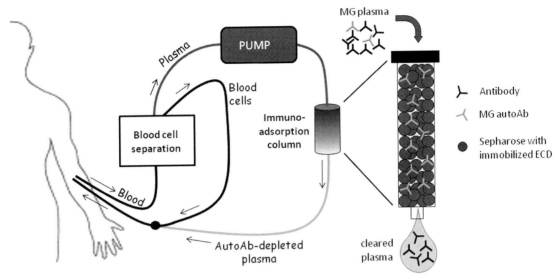

Figure 1. Schematic representation of the antigen-specific immunoadsorption approach. The ECDs of the AChR or MuSK are immobilized onto sepharose beads and packed into a column through which the patient's plasma passes, allowing the selective binding and removal of only the MG autoantibodies. The cleared autoantibody-depleted plasma is then returned to the patient.

a marked increase in the protein's solubility, expression yield, and even antigenicity, as it was capable of binding a larger percentage of anti-AChR antibodies than its wild-type counterpart. We then investigated similar mutations of the cys-loop in the other subunit ECDs as well.[27] In accordance with the findings for the γ-ECD, they also exhibited better yields and antigenicity.

Although the antigenicity of the expressed ECDs increased, there was still a significant proportion of anti-AChR antibodies that was not recognized by any of the ECDs. In fact, we estimate that with the current adsorbents the immunoadsorption would be efficient for approximately 30% of AChR-MG patients. We attempted to improve this by coexpressing all ECDs, or by expressing ECD concatamers (more than one ECD linked in tandem by a flexible peptide linker), aiming to create pentameric ECDs more closely matched to the native AChR. In parallel we expressed the above mutant ECDs and ECD concatamers in higher expression systems such as insect and mammalian cell lines. Neither the coexpressions nor the pentameric concatamers resulted in significantly improved binding. On the other hand, expression in higher systems was beneficial with respect to antigenicity, but the expression yield was considerably lower, and was deemed insufficient for the large-scale expressions required.

Current efforts are focused on the expression of the full-length receptor subunits in mammalian and insect cells. Although the expression yield is not expected to be comparable to that of the ECDs, we hope to achieve significantly better antibody-binding efficiencies.

Column characterization

Although efforts to improve the antigenicity of the adsorbent are ongoing, we have initiated addressing other aspects of the procedure, such as scaling-up, in order to verify the feasibility for clinical use. For these experiments the α1-ECD and β1-ECD are being used, as between them they bind the majority of autoantibodies and they show the best expression characteristics.

Initially, we focused on the capacity of the adsorbents for autoantibodies—that is, the amount of autoantibodies that can be removed by a given quantity of ECD adsorbent. Studies with the wild-type ECDs had shown that their capacity was satisfactory—1.5 nmol antibody per mg ECD for the α1-ECD and 5 nmol for the β1-ECD.[22,23] Interestingly, initial results from experiments using the mutant ECDs to test for their capacity show it is at least 10-fold higher. In effect, this would translate to 3–5 mg of protein being sufficient for the clearance of the plasma (3 L) from an average titer patient (~50 nM), a quantity that can be easily obtained. Furthermore, this suggests that the adsorbent immobilized onto a single column would be adequate for a therapeutic session without the need for its regeneration, as is the case for currently applied immunoadsorption protocols.

Another important parameter is the speed of immunoadsorption, which needs to take place fast, otherwise the time required for treatment would not be realistic. In small-scale batch experiments autoantibody binding was very fast, with just three to four minutes required to reach the maximum binding potential.[22,23] Currently, we are examining the speed of adsorption with larger scale columns, so as to better mimic the actual conditions. Indeed, it appears that a medium-sized column (10 mL bed volume) retains its binding efficiency at plasma flow speeds of up to 50 mL/min. It is reasonable to assume that the more relevant columns of 20–30 mL, which will be used for therapy, will be able to reach the desired speed of 100–125 mL/min. Future experiments with such columns will address this question.

The regeneration of the columns—that is, the elution of the bound antibodies after a therapeutic session—would allow them to be reused by the same patient, thus greatly decreasing the cost of treatment. A number of experiments are under way exploring this possibility, by assessing the number of regeneration cycles the adsorption matrix can undergo before it loses its binding efficiency. We are testing the possibility of adsorbent leaching from the matrix due to the low pH treatment required to elute the bound antibodies. Preliminary results support that incubation of the matrix with a low pH glycine buffer does not result in more adsorbent being released from the sepharose beads. Furthermore, examination of the immunoadsorption suggests that for up to four regeneration cycles the adsorbent retains most of its binding capacity, allowing its reuse. To test the stability of the column when in use, we are also examining the possibility of increased leaching of adsorbent from the matrix due to contact with the patient's plasma. It appears that even an overnight incubation of the sepharose beads with plasma has no effect on leaching of adsorbent from the matrix. The completion of this set of experiments will allow us to determine the optimal conditions for column recycling.

Safety aspects

In order to advance to the development of the procedure for clinical use, a number of safety aspects need to be addressed, such as the possibility of complement activation in the patients' blood due to the treatment, toxicity effects of the adsorbent, and safety of the procedure.

Complement activation may occur in patients undergoing immunoadsorption, which can lead to side effects such as fever, muscle pain, and vomiting.[28,29] Even though complement activation is unlikely in the case of antigen-specific immunoadsorption due to the minute amount of antibodies removed, this possibility needs to be assessed. To this end, the impact on complement activation in MG and normal sera treated through an ECD-sepharose column is being examined. Indeed, preliminary experiments using two MG sera and a healthy control showed no complement activation in any of the tested sera; the procedure will be repeated with a larger number of samples to verify these results.

In addition, the possible toxicity of the adsorbents needs to be evaluated. Therefore, we are currently working with Lewis rats injected i.v. with each of the adsorbents (α1-ECD or β1-ECD) or with only buffer as a control. The animals are thereafter observed checking their general health, body weight change, and food consumption. At the end of the observation period, blood samples are taken for full blood and biochemical tests, while the animals are killed and a gross necropsy is performed. Preliminary results from a limited number of animals so far showed no signs of toxicity due to the adsorbent, that is, all tests were the same between the ECD injected and control animals, while no organomegaly was observed during the necropsy. These tests will be completed with the minimum number of animals required to provide a statistically reliable result.

Finally, we are in the process of assessing the safety of the procedure using experimental rabbits. The animals will be immunized in order to develop anti-AChR antibodies and then subjected to immunoadsorption. The efficiency of the procedure will be assessed by measurement of the remaining anti-AChR antibodies, but most importantly, the health of the animals will be monitored for signs of adverse effects. The results from a small experiment using two rabbits are very promising; we thus anticipate no problems in larger scale experiments.

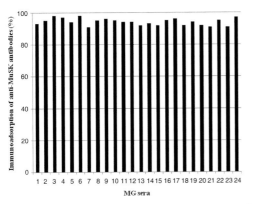

Figure 2. Immunoadsorption of MuSK-MG sera is practically complete. Screening of 24 MuSK-MG patients' sera for binding to MuSK-sepharose revealed the practically complete removal of all anti-MuSK antibodies from all sera. (From Trakas *et al.*[11])

MuSK as an immmunoadsorbent

Expression and characterization

The MuSK extracellular domain (MuSK-ECD) was expressed in the yeast *P. pastoris* and was found to be expressed as a soluble glycosylated polypeptide, with a yield of ~0.8 mg/L of cell culture.[11] Interestingly, when immobilized onto sepharose beads, in contrast to the AChR subunit adsorbents, it was found to bind 90–100% of anti-MuSK antibodies from all the patients' sera tested (Fig. 2). It therefore may be a very promising protein for use in immunoadsorption.

The further analysis of its characteristics as an adsorbent indicates that its capacity for autoantibodies is approximately 6 nmol/mg MuSK. Since the average titer of MuSK-MG patients is relatively low, 6 mg MuSK-ECD would be sufficient for the clearance of an average titer anti-MuSK plasma. On the other hand, ongoing work with respect to the recyclability suggests that the MuSK column appears to be more resistant to treatment with the low pH glycine buffer for elution of bound antibodies, being able to retain more than 80% of its capacity even after seven regeneration cycles.

Safety aspects

Similar to the AChR ECD adsorbents, a number of safety issues must be addressed before MuSK immunoadsorption can be considered for human use. We are in the process of assessing the safety of the procedure using experimental rabbits. Currently, the procedure is being studied in healthy (nonimmunized) rabbits, and initial observations show no pathological findings or adverse reactions. Subsequently, the animals will be immunized in order to develop autoantibodies and then treated with immunoadsorption. The efficiency of the procedure will be assessed by measurement of the remaining autoantibodies, while the health of the animals (body temperature and blood tests) will be observed for signs of adverse reactions. Furthermore, since it is likely that the immunized rabbits will also develop symptoms, it will be of great interest to see a reduction in the severity or even elimination of these symptoms altogether after the commencement of the immunoadsorptions.

Conclusions

The available data support that antigen-specific immunoadsorption can be a safe and efficient method of treatment for MG patients. Although there is still progress to be made with respect to the AChR ECD adsorbents, which currently work efficiently for only ~30% of patients, the MuSK-ECD adsorbent was shown to be very effective for all the sera tested.[11] Moreover, the adsorption appears to be fast and efficient, which paves the way for the treatment of the large volumes of patient plasma that will be required in practice. Initial data with respect to column regeneration at a large scale suggest that the columns can be regenerated, albeit for only a limited number of times in the case of the AChR ECD adsorbents, which could lead to the reduction of treatment costs. Finally, animal studies have so far shown no adverse reactions to either the adsorbents or the procedure itself. The successful completion of the safety tests and upscaling experiments is crucial for advancement into clinical trials. The apheresis strategy proposed here, if developed will be the first antigen-specific therapy for MG, and could act as a model for the development of similar therapies for other related autoimmune diseases as well.

Acknowledgments

This work was supported by Grants from the European Commission (FP7 Fight-MG, contract no. 242210; REGPOT NeuroSign, contract no. 264033), the Muscular Dystrophy Association (MDA), and the Association Francaise contre les Myopathies (AFM).

Conflicts of interest

Socrates Tzartos is coinventor in a patent that relates to immunoadsorption of anti-AChR autoantibodies (Patent no. EP 1509605/2009).

References

1. Meriggioli, M.N. & D.B. Sanders. 2009. Autoimmune myasthenia gravis: emerging clinical and biological heterogeneity. *Lancet Neurol.* **8:** 475–490.
2. Kalamida, D., K. Poulas, V. Avramopoulou, *et al.* 2007. Muscle and neuronal nicotinic acetylcholine receptors. Structure, function and pathogenicity. *FEBS J.* **274:** 3799–3845.
3. Tzartos, S.J. & J.M. Lindstrom. 1980. Monoclonal antibodies used to probe acetylcholine receptor structure: localization of the main immunogenic region and detection of similarities between subunits. *Proc. Natl. Acad. Sci. USA* **77:** 755–759.
4. Tzartos, S. J., T. Barkas, M.T. Cung, *et al.* 1998. Anatomy of the antigenic structure of a large membrane autoantigen, the muscle-type nicotinic acetylcholine receptor. *Immunol. Rev.* **163:** 89–120.
5. Luo, J., P. Taylor, M. Losen, *et al.* 2009. Main immunogenic region structure promotes binding of conformation-dependent myasthenia gravis autoantibodies, nicotinic acetylcholine receptor conformation maturation, and agonist sensitivity. *J. Neurosci.* **29:** 13898–13908.
6. Lindstrom, J.M., A.G. Engel, M.E. Seybold, *et al.* 1976. Pathological mechanisms in experimental autoimmune myasthenia gravis. II: passive transfer of experimental autoimmune myasthenia gravis in rats with anti-acetylcholine recepotr antibodies. *J. Exp. Med.* **144:** 739–753.
7. Newsom-Davis, J., S.G. Wilson, A. Vincent & C.D. Ward. 1979. Long-term effects of repeated plasma exchange in myasthenia gravis. *Lancet* **1:** 464–468.
8. Gomez, A.M., J. Van Den Broeck, K. Vrolix, *et al.* 2010. Antibody effector mechanisms in myasthenia gravis-pathogenesis at the neuromuscular junction. *Autoimmunity* **43:** 353–370.
9. Hoch, W., J. McConville, S. Helms, *et al.* 2001. Autoantibodies to the receptor tyrosine kinase MuSK in patients with myasthenia gravis without acetylcholine receptor antibodies. *Nat. Med.* **7:** 365–368.
10. Leite, M.I., S. Jacob, S. Viegas, *et al.* 2008. IgG1 antibodies to acetylcholine receptors in 'seronegative' myasthenia gravis. *Brain* **131:** 1940–1952.
11. Trakas, N., P. Zisimopoulou & S.J. Tzartos. 2011. Development of a highly sensitive diagnostic assay for muscle-specific tyrosine kinase (MuSK) autoantibodies in myasthenia gravis. *J. Neuroimmunol.* **240-241:** 79–86.
12. Higuchi, O., J. Hamuro, M. Motomura & Y. Yamanashi. 2011. Autoantibodies to low-density lipoprotein receptor-related protein 4 in myasthenia gravis. *Ann. Neurol.* **69:** 418–422.
13. Zhang, B., J.S. Tzartos, M. Belimezi, *et al.* 2012. Autoantibodies to lipoprotein-related protein 4 in patients with double-seronegative myasthenia gravis. *Arch. Neurol.* **69:** 445–451.
14. Pevzner, A., B. Schoser, K. Peters, *et al.* 2012. Anti-LRP4 autoantibodies in AChR- and MuSK-antibody-negative myasthenia gravis. *J. Neurol.* **259:** 427–435.
15. Sanders, D.B. & A. Evoli. 2010. Immunosuppressive therapies in myasthenia gravis. *Autoimmunity* **43:** 428–435.
16. Gilhus, N.E., J.F. Owe, J.M. Hoff, *et al.* 2011. Myasthenia gravis: a review of available treatment approaches. *Autoimmune Dis.* **2011:** 847393.
17. Matic, G., T. Bosch & W. Ramlow. 2001. Background and indications for protein A-based extracorporeal immunoadsorption. *Ther. Apher.* **5:** 394–403.
18. Ptak, J. 2004. Changes of plasma proteins after immunoadsorption using Ig-Adsopak columns in patients with myasthenia gravis. *Transfus. Apher. Sci.* **30:** 125–129.
19. Lagoumintzis, G., P. Zisimopoulou, K.G. Kordas, *et al.* 2010. Recent approaches to the development of antigen-specific immunotherapies for myasthenia gravis. *Autoimmunity* **43:** 1–10.
20. Psaridi-Linardaki, L., A. Mamalaki, M. Remoundos & S.J. Tzartos. 2002. Expression of soluble ligand- and antibody-binding extracellular domain of human muscle acetylcholine receptor alpha subunit in yeast Pichia pastoris. Role of glycosylation in alpha-bungarotoxin binding. *J. Biol. Chem.* **277:** 26980–26986.
21. Kostelidou, K., N. Trakas, M. Zouridakis, *et al.* 2006. Expression and characterization of soluble forms of the extracellular domains of the beta, gamma and epsilon subunits of the human muscle acetylcholine receptor. *FEBS J.* **273:** 3557–3568.
22. Psaridi-Linardaki, L., N. Trakas, A. Mamalaki & S.J. Tzartos. 2005. Specific immunoadsorption of the autoantibodies from myasthenic patients using the extracellular domain of the human muscle acetylcholine receptor alpha-subunit. Development of an antigen-specific therapeutic strategy. *J. Neuroimmunol.* **159:** 183–191.
23. Kostelidou, K., N. Trakas & S.J. Tzartos. 2007. Extracellular domains of the beta, gamma and epsilon subunits of the human acetylcholine receptor as immunoadsorbents for myasthenic autoantibodies: a combination of immunoadsorbents results in increased efficiency. *J. Neuroimmunol.* **190:** 44–52.
24. Sideris, S., G. Lagoumintzis, G. Kordas, *et al.* 2007. Isolation and functional characterization of anti-acetylcholine receptor subunit-specific autoantibodies from myasthenic patients: receptor loss in cell culture. *J. Neuroimmunol.* **189:** 111–117.
25. Zisimopoulou, P., G. Lagoumintzis, K. Poulas & S.J. Tzartos. 2008. Antigen-specific apheresis of human anti-acetylcholine receptor autoantibodies from myasthenia gravis patients' sera using Escherichia coli-expressed receptor domains. *J. Neuroimmunol.* **200:** 133–141.
26. Bitzopoulou, K., K. Kostelidou, K. Poulas & S.J. Tzartos. 2008. Mutant forms of the extracellular domain of the human acetylcholine receptor gamma-subunit with improved solubility and enhanced antigenicity. The importance of the Cys-loop. *Biochim. Biophys. Acta* **1784:** 1226–1233.
27. Zisimopoulou, P., G. Lagoumintzis, K. Kostelidou, *et al.* 2008. Towards antigen-specific apheresis of pathogenic autoantibodies as a further step in the treatment of myasthenia gravis by plasmapheresis. *J. Neuroimmunol.* **201-202:** 95–103.
28. Vamvakas, E.C. & A.A. Pineda. 1997. *Apheresis—Principle and Practice.* AABB Press. Bethesda, MD.
29. Ptak, J. & J. Lochman. 2005. Immunoadsorption therapy and complement activation. *Transfus. Apher. Sci.* **32:** 263–267.

Ann. N.Y. Acad. Sci. ISSN 0077-8923

Further developments with antisense treatment for myasthenia gravis

Jon Sussman,[1] Zohar Argov,[2] Yitzhak Wirguin,[3*] Slobodan Apolski,[4] Vedrana Milic-Rasic,[5] and Hermona Soreq[6]

[1]Greater Manchester Neuroscience Centre, Manchester UK. [2]Hadassah-Hebrew University Medical Centre, Jerusalem, Israel. [3]Soroka Medical Centre, Beer Sheva, Israel. [4]Institute of Neurology, University of Belgrade, Serbia. [5]Clinic for Neurology and Psychiatry, Belgrade, Serbia. [6]The Edmond and Lily Safra Center of Brain Science, The Hebrew University of Jerusalem, Israel 91904

Address for correspondence: Dr. Jon Sussman, Department of Neurology, Greater Manchester Neuroscience Centre, Hope Hospital, Stott Lane, Salford, Greater Manchester, UK, M6 8HD. jon.sussman@manchester.ac.uk

We present further developments in the study of the antisense oligonucleotide EN101. Ongoing *in vitro* and *in vivo* studies demonstrate that EN101 is a TLR9-specific ligand that can suppress pro-inflammatory functions and shift nuclear factor kappa B (NF-κB) from the pro-inflammatory canonical pathway to the anti-inflammatory alternative pathway, which results in decreases acetylcholinesterase (AChE) activity. Preliminary results of a double-blinded phase II cross-over study compared 10, 20, and 40 mg EN101 administered to patients with myasthenia gravis. Patients were randomly assigned to one of three treatment groups in weeks 1, 3, and 5 and received their pretreatment dose of pyridostigmine in weeks 2 and 4. Thus far, all doses show a decrease in QMG scores, with a greater response to higher doses.

Keywords: acetylcholinesterase; read-through transcript; antisense; TLR9

Introduction

Myasthenia gravis is a well-characterized neuromuscular autoimmune disease in which defective cholinergic transmission leads to weakness and fatigability of voluntary muscle. Neuromuscular synaptic functioning involves the nicotinic acetylcholine receptor (nAChR) and acetylcholinesterase (AChE), whose functions are closely interrelated. AChE hydrolyses acetylcholine (ACh), terminating neurotransmission. In humans, AChE is encoded by a single gene located on chromosome 7q22, but multiple splice variants arise from alternative splicing of exons at the 3′ end of the open reading frame. The principal transcript in muscle is the synaptic form AChE-S, in which exon 4 is spliced to exon 6. The read-through transcript AChE-R is a continuous transcript from exon 1 to exon 6, including intron 4.[1] Both forms of the enzyme hydrolyse acetylcholine,

AChE-S forms multimers and associates with the postsynaptic membrane, whereas AChE-R lacks the carboxyl-terminal cysteine that is required for binding and is a soluble monomer.[2–4] Rats with experimental autoimmune myasthenia gravis (EAMG) have increased blood levels of AChE-R. *In situ* hybridization shows markedly increased muscle staining for AChE-R mRNA but normal levels of AChE-S, suggesting selective overexpression of AChE-R. Serum from half of patients with myasthenia gravis contains AChE-R, which is not found in healthy humans.[5,6]

Mechanisms of action

The rationale for creating EN101 was as an antisense treatment designed to bind to AChE-R. In the development of the antisense, various oligonucleotides targeted to the AChE gene were tested, with EN101 being selected for greatest efficacy. In cell cultures, EN101 onset of action within 30–60 minutes is compatible with an antisense mode of action.[9,10]

---

*Deceased.

doi: 10.1111/j.1749-6632.2012.06825.x

Studies have shown that antisense and siRNA agents may exert nontarget-related biological effects including immunomodulation.[11] The rapid action, low effective dose, and long-lasting effects of EN101 raised the possibility that it might also have nonantisense properties. To challenge this prediction, EN101 was placed on HEK-293 cell lines expressing a range of Toll-like receptors (TLRs) and was shown to selectively stimulate the cell line expressing TLR9. Specific inhibitors of TLR9 and inhibitors of endosomal maturation blocked this effect, confirming the specificity of this binding. Also, there was no effect for EN101 in TLR9 knockout or MyD88 knockout animals, confirming that blocking the signaling pathway for the production of inflammatory cytokines prevented changes in TLR9 action under EN101.[12]

An association between AChE activity and TLR9 stimulation has been shown to be linked in murine and human mononuclear cells in culture; TLR9 agonism and a reduction in AChE activity is induced by EN101, and both effects are blocked by TLR9 inhibitors. In mouse mononuclear cells in culture, EN101 acts via the alternative TLR9 pathway.[12]

The interrelationship between cholinergic activity and cytokine production has been studied in the NOD mouse model of Sjögren's disease and *in vivo* using human Sjögren's disease salivary gland biopsies. Sjögren's disease in human biopsies and the murine model of the disease are associated with elevated IL-1b, and suppressed alternative NF-κB pathway markers. In the NOD mouse model, EN101 reduces AChE and inflammatory cytokine levels, increases saliva production, and increases alternative NF-κB pathway markers.[12]

The direct relevance of studies of Sjögren's disease to MG is unclear. The results suggest that a mechanism of action other than antisense may be active in MG and show a mechanistic relationship between reduced AChE and an anti-inflammatory effect that was previously suggested in intact monkey spinal cord exposed to EN101.[13] The site of action of such effect in MG is speculative and might involve any part of the immune system, particularly the enteric immune system that might initially be exposed to an oral agent.

Animal studies

In order to investigate the role of AChE-R *in vivo* in rats with EAMG, an antisense oligonucleotide was designed to target and selectively destroy AChE-R. Antisense oligonucleotides are short synthetic stands of modified DNA or RNA designed to hybridise with target-specific mRNA by Watson–Crick base pairing. Binding activates RNAses that degrade the mRNA-antisense complex, thereby blocking synthesis of the protein encoded by the mRNA sequence. The antisense EN101 is a 20-mer oligonucleotide, modified by incorporating 2-*O*-methyl groups in the last three nucleotides at its 3′ end, which protects it from nucleolytic degradation. EN101 binds to a coding sequence common to all isoforms of AChE. The AChE-R mRNA transcript is intrinsically less stable and more sensitive to EN101, which was shown to be active both intravenously and orally.[5,7]

EN101 administration to EAMG rats results in a significant reduction in muscle AChE-R without any significant reduction in AChE-S. Neurophysiology studies of EAMG rats showed decrement during repeated nerve stimulation that is reversed by EN101. The rats have significantly improved ambulation and stamina when tested on a treadmill, and improved survival.[5]

Human studies

Phase Ib study

We previously published a phase Ib, nonplacebo controlled, open-label study[8] of oral EN101 in 16 patients with seropositive MG. Doses were derived from the efficacy studies performed in rats with EAMG. The dose was titrated up until a clinical response was detected. On day 1, patients received a single dose of 10 μg/kg, followed four hours later by 50 μg/kg, and a further four hours later by 150 μg/kg. Then, for three consecutive days the patients received a single dose of 500 μg/kg in the morning. The patients were assessed using the QMG score. The baseline QMG score was 14.9 (± 7.25). Thirteen of the 15 patients (87%) had improvement in QMG score on day 4 compared with baseline. The overall mean change of the QMG score from baseline was 6.13 (± 4.5) and the overall mean percent improvement from baseline was 46.5%. The EN101 antisense molecule given orally was well tolerated with no major adverse events and, of note, absence of cholinergic side effects.[8] Ethical and practical difficulties limit the use of placebo-controlled blinded studies in MG patients. The phase Ib safety study had therefore been designed primarily as an open-label safety study. The results suggested that low-dose EN101 had statistically significant but modest efficacy, which had not been apparent during the dose titration phase of the study.

Current phase II study

We have followed that work with a phase II study of efficacy designed to blindly compare three doses of EN101. The study is designed to compare QMG following treatment with 10, 20, and 40 mg doses of EN101, each administered for seven days, with one week of treatment with pyridostigmine between each period on EN101. The entry criteria to the study include seropositive myasthenia gravis with AChR antibodies, a minimum severity of MGFA class II, and the demonstration of response to pyridostigmine, as determined by worsening of at least 3 points on the QMG scale on its withdrawal. Exclusion criteria include administration of IVIg or plasma exchange in the previous two months. As the intention is to compare three doses of EN101 blindly, the pyridostigmine dose is not altered from the dose used previously during routine treatment. Safety is assessed by evaluating adverse events and laboratory tests during five weeks, and after a four-week follow-up period.

Preliminary results from the study carried out in six centers, two each in UK, Israel, and Serbia, include data on 31 patients. The mean age is 55.9 years, and there are 21 males and 11 females. The mean duration of MG is 9.9 years. Of the 31 patients, 8 discontinued after screening. A significant worsening in MG was defined as an adverse event, and a number of patients withdrew between screening and commencing the study or became unwell with intercurrent illnesses during the study. None occurred while receiving EN101. A total of 23 completed the study; of those one mistakenly took pyridostigmine and thereby failed to follow the protocol. One patient died of a cerebral hemorrhage while taking pyridostigmine between the second and third week of EN101. She had longstanding diabetes and hypertension. Her death was not thought to be connected with the trial. A total of 22 completed the protocol.

Thus far the study has demonstrated deterioration on withdrawal from pyridostigmine at screening, with improvement in QMG score following each seven-day treatment with EN101. All doses have demonstrated efficacy compared with baseline QMG score; however, there is no statistically significant difference between the three doses, though there is a trend toward a dose response. The lowest effective dose and maximum response to EN101 have not been identified. Adverse events that might be associated with EN101 treatment were few, with complaint of a dry mouth affecting a maximum of 6.7%, and headache 7.1%. Adverse events were not related to dose. Four serious adverse events were reported during the ITT study. None were thought to be related to EN101, and none occurred while taking EN101. There were no complaints of abdominal cramps or diarrhea.

Conclusions

Two studies have thus far shown that EN101 has efficacy in the treatment of MG without cholinergic side effects, although the optimal dose remains uncertain. No direct comparison of efficacy of pyridostigmine and EN101 has been performed; in the phase II study in which the dose of pyridostigmine is not optimized, EN101 appears to have greater efficacy. The potential of this drug in everyday treatment remains unclear, however. EN101 undoubtedly has fewer side effects than pyridostigmine so it may have a role as a symptomatic treatment. A rapid onset of efficacy shown to be four hours in the phase I study with an improvement on the QMG scale of 6.13 ± 4.5 points after 96 hours raises the potential for a role in the management of acute relapses. The duration of action of EN101 is uncertain—the open-label one-month follow-up study following the phase I study demonstrated continuing efficacy; however it is unclear whether it could be used for long-term treatment. The mechanisms of action appear fortuitously to combine a reduction in AChE production with an immunomodulatory role. The relative contribution of each function is unclear; however the immunomodulatory potential of EN101 would justify future trials into its efficacy as a steroid sparing agent and whether it might take the place of immunosuppressive drugs.

Conflicts of interest

The authors declare no conflicts of interest.

References

1. Li, Y., S. Camp, T.L. Rachinsky, *et al.* 1991. Gene structure of mammalian acetylcholinesterase. Alternative exons dictate tissue-specific expression. *J. Biol. Chem.* **266:** 23083–23090.

2. Grisaru, D., M. Sternfeld, A. Eldor, *et al.* 1999. Structural roles of acetylcholinesterase variants in biology and pathology. *Eur. J. Biochem.* **264:** 672–686.

3. Seidman, S., M., Sternfeld, R. Ben Aziz-Aloya, *et al.* 1995. Synaptic and epidermal accumulations of human acetylcholinesterase are encoded by alternative 3′-terminal exons. *Mol. Cell. Biol.* **15:** 2993–3002.

4. Soreq, H. & S. Seidman. 2001. Acetylcholinesterase—new roles for an old actor. *Nat. Neurosci. Rev.* **2:** 294–302.

5. Brenner, T., Y. Hamra-Amitay, T. Evron, *et al.* 2003. The role of readthrough acetylcholinesterase in the pathophysiology of myasthenia gravis. *FASEB J.* **17:** 214–222.

6. Boneva, N., Y. Hamra-Amitay, I. Wiruin, *et al.* 2006. Stimulated-single fiber electromyography monitoring of anti-sense induced changes in experimental autoimmune myasthenia gravis. *Neurosci. Res.* **55:** 40–44.

7. Pollak, Y., A. Gilboa, O. Ben-Menachem, *et al.* 2005. Acetylcholinesterase modulates interleukin-1β production in the hippocampus and blood. *Ann. Neurol.* **57:** 741–745.

8. Argov, Z., D. McKee, S. Agus, *et al.* 2007. Treatment of human myasthenia gravis with oral antisense suppression of acetylcholinesterase. *Neurology* **69:** 699–700.

9. Grifman, M. & H. Soreq. 1997. Differentiation intensifies the susceptibility of phaeochromocytoma cells to antisense oligodeoxynucleotide-dependent suppression of acetylcholinesterase activity. *Antisense Res. Nucleic Acids Drug Dev.* **7:** 351–359.

10. Galyam, N., D. Grisaru, N. Melamed-Book, *et al.* 2001. Complex host cell responses to antisense suppression of ACHE gene expression. *Antisense Nucleic Acid Drug Dev.* **11:** 51–57.

11. Agrawal S. & E.R. Kandimalla. 2004. Role of Toll-like receptors in antisense and siRNA. *Nat. Biotechnol.* **22:** 1533–7. *Erratum in Nat. Biotechnol.* 2005 Jan; **23**(1): 117.

12. Gilboa-Geffen A., Y. Wolf, G. Hanin, *et al.* 2011. Activation of the alternative NFκB pathway improves disease symptoms in a model of Sjögren's syndrome. *PLoS One* **6:** e28727.

13. Evron, T., L. Ben-Moyal, N. Lam, *et al.* 2005. RNA-targeted suppression of stress-induced allostasis in monkey spinal cord neurons. *Neurodegenerat. Dis.* **2:** 16–27.

Ann. N.Y. Acad. Sci. ISSN 0077-8923

ANNALS OF THE NEW YORK ACADEMY OF SCIENCES

Issue: *Myasthenia Gravis and Related Disorders*

Design of the Efficacy of Prednisone in the Treatment of Ocular Myasthenia (EPITOME) trial

Michael Benatar,[1] Donald B. Sanders,[2] Gil I. Wolfe,[3] Michael P. McDermott,[4,5] and Rabi Tawil[5]

[1]Department of Neurology, University of Miami, Miller School of Medicine, Miami, Florida. [2]Division of Neurology, Department of Medicine, Duke University, Durham, North Carolina. [3]Department of Neurology, University at Buffalo School of Medicine and Biomedical Sciences, State University of New York, Buffalo, New York. [4]Department of Biostatistics and Computational Biology, University of Rochester Medical Center, Rochester, New York. [5]Department of Neurology, University of Rochester Medical Center, Rochester, New York

Address for correspondence: Michael Benatar, MBChB, MS, DPhil, Department of Neurology, University of Miami, Clinical Research Building, Room 1318, 1120 NW 14th Street, Miami, FL, 33136. mbenatar@med.miami.edu

Efficacy of Prednisone in the Treatment of Ocular Myasthenia (EPITOME) is a multicenter, randomized, double blind, placebo-controlled trial that is being conducted under the auspices of the Muscle Study Group. EPITOME is the first randomized control trial in patients with ocular myasthenia and aims to evaluate the efficacy and tolerability of prednisone over a period of four months in patients with newly diagnosed ocular myasthenia whose symptoms have failed to remit in response to a trial of cholinesterase inhibitor therapy.

Keywords: ocular myasthenia; steroids; clinical trial; evidence-based medicine

Introduction

Myasthenia gravis is a generalized disorder that often manifests initially as focal weakness. The most common focal presentation is ocular, with weakness involving the extraocular muscles, eyelid levators, and orbicularis oculi. The two leading ocular symptoms are ptosis and diplopia. The estimated prevalence of myasthenia gravis is ~10 per 100,000, with approximately 60% of patients initially presenting with isolated ocular symptoms.[1] About half of these patients will progress to develop generalized myasthenia gravis,[2–4] while the disease will remain purely ocular in the other half (~30% of all patients).[2,5–10]

The goals of treatment for ocular myasthenia (OM) are to return the person to a state of clear vision and to prevent the development or limit the severity of generalized myasthenia gravis (GMG). Treatments proposed for OM include drugs with a purely symptomatic effect such as cholinesterase inhibitors, as well as drugs that suppress the immune system such as corticosteroids. Proponents of steroids point to the limited efficacy of pyridostigmine, the potentially greater symptomatic effects of prednisone and the potential for steroids to reduce the risk of progression from ocular to generalized disease. Opponents emphasize the potential risk of serious side effects and question whether these risks are justified by the severity of, and functional limitations imposed by purely ocular symptoms.

There have been two prior randomized controlled trials (RCTs) relevant to the treatment of OM.[11,12] Neither trial permits any conclusion regarding the relative efficacy of cholinesterase inhibitor and steroid therapy. There have also been six nonrandomized observational studies,[13–17,18] four of which suggest a possible benefit of steroids with respect to reducing the risk of progression to GMG,[13–15,17] and one of which suggested a favorable symptomatic effect.[18] However, in view of the paucity and limited methodological quality of the available data, significant controversy persists regarding the optimal approach to the treatment of patients with OM.[19–21] The importance of the clinical question, combined with the equipoise among neuromuscular specialists and within the broader medical community, provides justification for an RCT comparing cholinesterase inhibitor therapy to the combination of steroids and a cholinesterase inhibitor. A practice parameter published by the

American Academy of Neurology concurred with the need for a well-designed, randomized, placebo-controlled study of the efficacy of cholinesterase inhibitors and corticosteroids in OM.[12]

Trial design

Overview

The EPITOME study is a randomized, double-blind, placebo-controlled trial that aims to address the equipoise that currently exists regarding the use of corticosteroids for treating patients with OM (Fig. 1). Prior to randomization all study participants are treated with pyridostigmine, which is titrated to efficacy or tolerability over four to six weeks. Participants whose symptoms fail to remit are randomized to receive either prednisone or placebo in a double-blind manner. The trial evaluates a prednisone dosing strategy—start low and titrate upward as needed based on efficacy and safety/tolerability—rather than a fixed dosage of prednisone. This dosing strategy was favored over the "start high and taper down" strategy because of concern for a greater risk for steroid side effects with the latter. Budgetary (and hence sample size) constraints precluded a three-arm trial, comparing both dosing strategies to placebo. Both groups are maintained on a stable dosage of pyridostigmine throughout the trial. After four months (stage 1), participants who fail to attain sustained minimal manifestation status (MMS) and do not experience dose-limiting adverse events will receive high-dosage prednisone with subsequent taper in an open-label fashion. Those who do achieve sustained MMS will have study drug tapered in a double-blind fashion (stage 2). The schedule of assessments during stage 2 mimics that of stage 1 in order to provide hypothesis-generating data about the relative safety and efficacy of the two different steroid dosing strategies.

Patient population

The trial eligibility criteria aim to enroll a sample of patients with new or recent onset of ocular myasthenia (< two years since symptom onset) who have not previously received immune suppressive or modulating therapy and who have not already received treatment with prednisone. Ocular myasthenia is defined, according to the Myasthenia Gravis Foundation of America (MGFA), as weakness due to myasthenia gravis that is limited to the extraocular muscles, the eyelid levators, and orbicularis oculi.[22] Inclusion criteria require some supplementary evidence to support the diagnosis (e.g., elevated acetylcholine receptor antibody titers, relevant abnormalities on repetitive nerve stimulation, or measurement of neuromuscular jitter).

Study drug

Prednisone will be started at a dosage of 10 mg every other day, with the dosage increased by 10 mg every two weeks; the dosage is initially increased to 10 mg/day, then 20 mg alternating with 10 mg, and so forth. The maximum dosage allowed during stage 1 is 40 mg/day. The dosage is titrated according to whether MMS has been attained and the presence and nature of adverse events. Dosage escalation is constrained by toxicity that does not respond to appropriate medical intervention. Open-label high-dosage prednisone is initiated at 60 mg/day in those who fail to achieve MMS during the double-blind phase and who have not already developed dose-limiting side effects; the dosage is quickly tapered based on efficacy and safety/tolerability.

Trial duration

The chosen four-month duration of the double-blind treatment period was felt to be sufficient to demonstrate the efficacy of prednisone in mitigating the symptoms of OM. A significantly longer duration of therapy would be needed to adequately evaluate the impact of steroids on the risk of progression to generalized disease, but this would also have entailed use of placebo over a substantially longer period of time. Four months was also deemed sufficient to detect most steroid-related side effects, although it is recognized that others might not evolve over this time period.

Outcome measures

The primary efficacy outcome measure will be treatment failure, defined as failure to achieve sustained MMS within four months of therapy, progression to GMG, or toxicity leading to discontinuation of study drug. This outcome is useful because it combines measures of efficacy and tolerability, and is clinically meaningful because it regards as treatment failures those whose symptoms do not remit within the four-month time frame of follow-up. MMS is regarded as sustained when it is observed at two consecutive in-person evaluations approximately one month apart. Sustained MMS is used instead of simply attainment

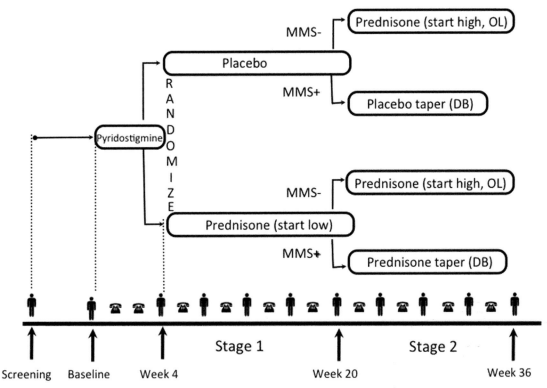

Figure 1. Trial schema. Potentially eligible trial participants are identified at screening and final eligibility determined using an evaluation of pyridostigmine at baseline. Pyridostigmine dosage is titrated to maximum efficacy and tolerability during the first four weeks of the trial. Those participants whose symptoms fail to remit are randomized at week 4 to receive either prednisone or placebo, at an initial starting dosage of 10 mg every other day. Monthly in-person evaluations and intervening telephone evaluations are used to titrate the dosage of prednisone on the basis of efficacy, tolerability, and safety. The study drug may be tapered in a double-blind fashion if participants achieve sustained MMS during stage1. Participants who first achieve minimal manifestation status (MMS+) by week 20 undergo a double-blind (DB) taper of study drug during stage 2 of the trial. Participants who do not achieve minimal manifestation status (MMS−) by week 20 and who have not experienced dose-limiting adverse events during stage 1 will be assigned open-label (OL) high-dosage (60 mg/day) prednisone during stage 2. The prednisone dosage is tapered during stage 2 on the basis of efficacy, safety, and tolerability. The final study visit occurs at week 36.

of MMS since the goal is to identify a durable treatment effect and to avoid declaring treatment success based simply on a temporary fluctuation in disease severity. Progression to GMG is defined on the basis of the results of MG-manual muscle testing (MG-MMT)[23] but also considers symptoms of dysphagia and dyspnea since these are not captured by the MG-MMT.

Secondary goals are to separately examine efficacy and safety/tolerability outcomes. For efficacy, we consider the time to sustained MMS, the time to an ocular Quantitative Myasthenia Gravis (QMG) score[18] of zero, and health-related quality of life (QoL) using the 25-item National Eye Institute Visual Function Questionnaire (VFQ-25),[24] the VFQ-25 10-item neuro-ophthalmological supplement,[25]

and the MG-QoL-15.[26] The ocular-QMG is based on the three ocular components of the QMG (ptosis, diplopia, and eye closure), but the diplopia component is expanded to include left gaze, right gaze, and upgaze. For the components of ptosis and diplopia (or restricted ocular motility), scores are assigned based on the latency to onset of symptoms—a score of 0 if symptoms do not emerge within 45 s, a score of 1 if symptoms emerge within 11–45 s, a score of 2 if symptoms emerge within 1–10 s, and a score of 3 if symptoms are spontaneous. Eye closure is scored as it is in the QMG.

For safety/tolerability, we will document study drug discontinuation, subject withdrawal, and individual adverse events. Active screening is employed to identify steroid-related adverse events. The impact of steroids on glycemic control is evaluated using glucose tolerance tests (nondiabetics) and glycosylated hemoglobin studies (diabetics) prior to treatment and at select intervals throughout the course of the trial. Dual energy X-ray absorptiometry (DEXA), bone density scans are performed at pre- and posttreatment time points, with prophylaxis against steroid-induced bone loss provided to all participants with reduced bone mineral density (t score < -1.0 in hip, femur, or spine). Pre- and posttreatment ophthalmological examinations are also performed to identify the emergence of glaucoma and cataracts.

Masking outcome measure assessment

All study personnel, other than personnel who generate the randomization plan and who package and label the study medication, will be blinded to treatment allocation. However, since the process of evaluating and managing adverse events may unmask the neurologist to the assigned treatment, the study design requires different assessments from two independent investigators. One investigator, designated as the treating neurologist, collects, reviews, and adjudicates adverse event data. The second investigator, designated as the blinded evaluator, will be responsible for determining the MGFA postintervention status (to ascertain the presence or absence of minimal manifestation status), and for performing the neuromuscular examination to evaluate whether there has been progression to GMG. The blinded evaluator will not participate in adverse event evaluations and study participants are specifically instructed to not communicate any adverse event data to the blinded evaluator. Questionnaires are administered to ascertain the success of these blinding procedures.

Cholinesterase inhibitor therapy

The ocular-QMG and MG-MMT are completed twice at the week four visit prior to randomization. The first set of evaluations is performed off pyridostigmine to ensure that the participant has not developed generalized MG that might otherwise be masked by symptomatic therapy with a cholinesterase inhibitor. The second set of evaluations is performed on pyridostigmine (within a 30- to 90-min time window of drug ingestion) to confirm that the participant has not attained MMS through the sole use of cholinesterase inhibitor therapy. Outcome measures at subsequent study visits

are performed on pyridostigmine because the study aims to compare the efficacy of pyridostigmine with that of the combination of prednisone and pyridostigmine.

Sample size considerations

Published retrospective data were used to estimate the sample size for the EPITOME trial. These data suggest that ~75% of OM patients achieve remission on prednisone plus pyridostigmine (after failing to remit on pyridostigmine alone), compared to 31% on pyridostigmine alone[18] over a four-month period. Key assumptions underlying our calculations include (a) some proportion (less than the observed 75%) of the prednisone treated group will achieve remission (i.e., $\geq$ 25% will experience treatment failure); (b) some proportion (less than the observed 31%) of the placebo treated group will remit (i.e., $\geq$ 69% will fail); and (c) prednisone will be stopped in ~10% of participants because of adverse events (this did not occur in our retrospective study). Based on (a) and (c), we assumed that $\geq$ 35% ($\geq$ 25% + 10%) of subjects in the prednisone group would experience treatment failure. A conclusion, based on these assumptions, is that a total sample size of 80 subjects (40 per group) will provide at least 80% power to detect absolute group differences of 30–35% using a chi-square test and a 5% significance level, as long as the proportion of treatment failures in the placebo group is at least 75%. A total sample size of 88 subjects will be enrolled in the trial to account for a projected loss to follow-up rate of $\leq$ 10%.

Discussion

The EPITOME trial was designed to mimic clinical practice to the greatest extent possible in order to ensure that the trial answers a clinically relevant question that can be generalized to a broad population of OM patients. For example, the trial is not limited to patients with acetylcholine receptor antibody positive disease. Similarly, patients with medical comorbidities that make the use of steroids challenging (e.g., patients with diabetes or osteoporosis) are not excluded as these are anticipated to be common medical problems within the potentially eligible study population. Moreover, the therapeutic approach is consistent with the dictates of clinical practice. For example, treatment begins with cholinesterase inhibitor therapy, and only those individuals who fail to adequately respond become eligible for randomization. The trial evaluates a steroid-dosing strategy rather than a fixed dosage of prednisone given the expectation, based on clinical experience, that different patients have varying steroid requirements. The dosage is titrated upward if symptoms persist in the absence of side effects and the dosage is tapered if side effects develop or if sustained MMS is achieved. The steroid-dosing strategy, therefore, aims to identify the minimum effective dosage that does not produce unacceptable side effects. In addition, the trial employs a fairly aggressive strategy for prospectively identifying potential steroid side effects, including glucose intolerance, reduced bone mineral density, cataracts, and glaucoma. To minimize the potential that review of steroid side effects will unmask the investigator to the treatment arm and thus bias outcome assessment, a treating neurologist will evaluate adverse event data, while a blinded evaluator assesses efficacy outcomes.

Although designed prior to publication of the recent MGFA recommendations for myasthenia gravis clinical trials,[27] EPITOME was developed with many of the same issues in mind. Already noted are the broad inclusion criteria, the aggressive monitoring for steroid side effects, and optimization of cholinesterase therapy prior to randomization. In addition, the number of trial sites has been doubled to 10 from the initial 5 to mitigate the risk of slow recruitment, and efforts are underway to incorporate a biomarker component into the trial.

Acknowledgments

We are grateful to the many people who have contributed to the design and implementation of this trial. Alexis Smirnow, Colleen Donlin-Smith, and Farheen Hussain have served as initial, interim, and current project managers, respectively, for the trial. Alexandre Waltz has overseen trial initiation at the University of Miami and Khema Sharma, MD serves as the blinded evaluator. The site investigators and their staff: Richard Barohn MD, Mamatha Pasnoor MD, Mazen Dimachkie MD, Yunxia Wang MD, Thomas Whittaker MD, Laura Herbelin, and Joseph Sibinski (Kansas University Medical Center); Srikanth Muppidi MD, Jaya Trivedi MD, and Nina Gorham CCRP (University of Texas Southwestern); Ted Burns MD, Guillermo Solorzano MD, Lawrence Phillips MD, Kelly Gwathmey MD, Raam Samban- dam MD, and Amruta Joshi MS, CRC (University of Virginia); Vern Juel MD, Jeffrey Guptill MD, Lisa Hobson-Webb MD, Janice Massey MD and Katherine Beck (Duke University); Michael Hehir MD, Rup Tandan MD, Waqar Waheed MD, and Shannon Lucy (University of Vermont). Randall Yeates and William Wilson at the University of Iowa Research Pharmacy for preparing study drug and matching placebo. Cornelia Kamp, Pat Bolger, Tim Hackett, and Joan Woodcook at the Clinical Material Services Unit (CMSU) at the University of Rochester, which serves as the central pharmacy for the trial. Joanne Janciuras at the University of Rochester who is the biostatistical programmer for the trial. Members of the Data and Safety Monitoring Board: Matthew Meriggioli MD (Chair), John Kissel MD, and Gary Cutter PhD, and Gregory Martin MD who serves as the Independent Medical Monitor.

Conflicts of interest

The authors declare no conflicts of interest.

References

1. Ferguson, F.R., E.C. Hutchinson & L.A. Liversedge. 1955. Myasthenia gravis; results of medical management. *Lancet* **269:** 636–639.
2. Robertson, N., J. Deans & D. Compston. 1998. Myasthenia gravis: a population based epidemiological study in Cambridgeshire, England. *J. Neurol. Neurosurg. Psychiatr.* **65:** 492–6.
3. Weizer, J.S., A.G. Lee & D.K. Coats. 2001. Myasthenia gravis with ocular involvement in older patients. *Can. J. Ophthalmol.* **36:** 26–33.
4. Bever, C.T., A.V. Aquino, A.S. Penn, *et al.* 1983. Prognosis of ocular myasthenia. *Ann. Neurol.* **14:** 516–519.
5. Christensen, P.B., T.S. Jensen, I. Tsiropoulos, *et al.* 1993. Incidence and prevalence of myasthenia gravis in western Denmark: 1975 to 1989. *Neurology* **43:** 1779–1783.
6. Casetta, I., E. Fallica, V. Govoni, *et al.* 2004. Incidence of myasthenia gravis in the province of Ferrara: a community-based study. *Neuroepidemiology* **23:** 281–284.
7. Lavrnic, D., M. Jarebinski, Rakocevic-Stojanovic V, *et al.* 1999. Epidemiological and clinical characteristics of myasthenia gravis in Belgrade, Yugoslavia (1983–1992). *Acta Neurologica Scandinavica* **100:** 168–174.
8. Phillips, L.H., J.C. Torner, M.S. Anderson & G.M. Cox. 1992. The epidemiology of myasthenia gravis in central and western Virginia. *Neurology* **42:** 1888–1893.
9. anonymous. 1998. Incidence of myasthenia gravis in the Emilia-Romagna region: a prospective multicenter study. Emilia-Romagna Study Group on Clinical and Epidemiological Problems in Neurology. *Neurology* **51:** 255–258.
10. Aiello, I., M. Pastorino, S. Sotgiu, *et al.* 1997. Epidemiology of myasthenia gravis in northwestern Sardinia. *Neuroepidemiol.* **16:** 199–206.

11. Benatar, M. & H. Kaminski. 2006. Medical and surgical treatments for ocular myasthenia. *Cochrane Database Syst. Rev.* Apr. **19;** (2): CD005081.

12. Benatar, M. & H.J. Kaminski. 2007. Evidence report: the medical treatment of ocular myasthenia (an evidence-based review): report of the Quality Standards Subcommittee of the American Academy of Neurology. *Neurology* **68:** 2144–2149.

13. Kupersmith, M.J., R. Latkany & P. Homel. 2003. Development of generalized disease at 2 years in patients with ocular myasthenia gravis. *Arch. Neurol.* **60:** 243–248.

14. Mee, J., M. Paine, E. Byrne, *et al.* 2003. Immunotherapy of ocular myasthenia gravis reduces conversion to generalized myasthenia gravis. *J. Neuroophthalmol.* **23:** 251–255.

15. Monsul, N.T., H.S. Patwa, A.M. Knorr, *et al.* 2004. The effect of prednisone on the progression from ocular to generalized myasthenia gravis. *J. Neurol. Sci.* **217:** 131–133.

16. Papapetropoulos, T.H., J. Ellul & E. Tsibri. 2003. Development of generalized myasthenia gravis in patients with ocular myasthenia gravis. *Arch. Neurol.* **60:** 1491–1492.

17. Sommer, N., B. Sigg, A. Melms, *et al.* 1997. Ocular myasthenia gravis: response to long-term immunosuppressant treatment. *J. Neurol. Neurosurg. Psychiatr.* **62:** 156–162.

18. Bhanushali, M., J. Wuu & M. Benatar. 2008. Treatment of ocular myasthenia. *Neurology* **71:** 1335–1341.

19. Agius M. 2000. Treatment of ocular myasthenia with corticosteroids: yes. *Arch. Neurol.* **57:** 750–751.

20. Hachinski V. 2000. Treatment of ocular myasthenia. *Arch. Neurol.* **57:** 753.

21. Kaminski, H. & R. Daroff. 2000. Treatment of ocular myasthenia: steroids only when compelled. *Arch. Neurol.* **57:** 752–753.

22. Jaretzki, A., R. Barohn, R. Ernstoff, *et al.* 2000. Myasthenia gravis: recommendations for clinical research standards. Task Force of the Medical Scientific Advisory Board of the Myasthenia Gravis Foundation of America. *Neurology* **55:** 16–23.

23. Sanders, D.B., B. Tucker-Lipscomb & J.M. Massey. 2003. A simple manual muscle test for myasthenia gravis: validation and comparison with the QMG score. *Ann. N.Y. Acad. Sci.* **998:** 440–444.

24. Mangione, C.M., P.P. Lee, P.R. Gutierrez, *et al.* 2001. Development of the 25-item National Eye Institute Visual Function Questionnaire. *Arch. Ophthalmol.* **119:** 1050–1058.

25. Raphael, B.A., K.M. Galetta, D.A. Jacobs, *et al.* 2006. Validation and test characteristics of a 10-item neuro-ophthalmic supplement to the NEI-VFQ-25. *Am. J. Ophthalmol.* **142:** 1026–1035.

26. Burns, T.M., M.R. Conaway, G.R. Cutter & D.B. Sanders. 2008. Less is more, or almost as much: a 15-item quality-of-life instrument for myasthenia gravis. *Muscle Nerve* **38:** 957–963.

27. Benatar, M., D.B. Sanders, T.M. Burns, *et al.* 2012. Recommendations for myasthenia gravis clinical trials. *Muscle Nerve* **45:** 909–917.

Ann. N.Y. Acad. Sci. ISSN 0077-8923

Phase II trial of methotrexate in myasthenia gravis

Mamatha Pasnoor, Jianghua He, Laura Herbelin, Mazen Dimachkie, Richard J. Barohn, and the Muscle Study Group

University of Kansas Medical Center, Kansas City, Kansas

Address for correspondence: Mamatha Pasnoor, University of Kansas Medical Center, 3901 Rainbow Blvd/MSN2012, Kansas City, KS 66160. mpasnoor@kumc.edu

Prednisone is a frequently used treatment for myasthenia gravis (MG) but it has numerous side effects. Methotrexate is a selective inhibitor of dihydrofolate reductase and lymphocyte proliferation and is an effective immuosuppressive medication for autoimmune diseases. Given the negative results of the mycophenolate mofetil study, search for an effective immunosuppressant drug therapy is ongoing. The objective is to determine if oral methotrexate is safe and effective for MG patients who take prednisone. We have initiated a randomized, double-blind, placebo-controlled multicenter trial of methotrexate versus placebo in patients taking at least 10 mg/day of prednisone at enrollment. The methotrexate dose is increased to 20 mg and the prednisone dose is adjusted per protocol during the study. Clinical and laboratory evaluations are performed monthly for 12 months, with the primary efficacy measure being the nine-month prednisone area under the curve (AUC) from months 3 to 12. Secondary outcome measures include MG outcomes, quality of life measures, and a polyglutamation biomarker assay. A total of 18 U.S. sites and 2 Canadian sites are participating, with 48 screened cases, 42 enrolled, with 19 still active in the study.

Keywords: methotrexate; myasthenia gravis; area under the curve; prednisone

Introduction

A number of attempts have been made to suppress the immune system and the associated antibody response in myasthenia gravis (MG). Thymectomy was first performed more than a half-century ago and was the earliest form of immune-directed therapy in MG. The introduction of corticosteroids in the therapy of MG was a major clinical advance. However, corticosteroids can have dose-limiting side effects, such as generalized immunosuppression, hyperglycemia, hypertension, myopathy, weight gain, cataracts, and osteoporosis. Other approaches to immunosuppression have come into clinical use in recent years. Recently two multicenter controlled trials of mycophenolate mofetil showed no benefit in MG.[1–4] These disappointing findings have prompted interest in looking for other immunosuppressive drugs that are currently available and have led to our interest in methotrexate (MTX) for MG. The potential advantages of MTX include oral dosing once a week, a relative moderate side effect profile, inexpensive cost, easy availability, availability in a generic oral preparation, and potential use for longer periods of time.

Methotrexate has been used and shown to be effective for autoimmune disorders such as rheumatoid arthritis[5–12] and multiple sclerosis.[13–15] Abdou *et al.* reported a small open-label series of MG patients who received 25–50 mg of MTX intramuscular weekly for up to 20 months; 87% showed some improvement.[16] In a small retrospective study of 16 patients, Hartmann showed improvement in 6 patients on MTX.[17] Recently, Heckmann *et al.* performed a single-blinded trial of MTX versus azathioprine as steroid-sparing agents in generalized myasthenia gravis and showed that MTX is an effective steroid-sparing agent 10 months after treatment initiation and that MTX has similar efficacy and tolerability to azathioprine.[18] A small retrospective study by Raja at the University of Kansas Medical Center in 2009 looked at eight MG patients on MTX, two showed improvement and prednisone dose was decreased in four patients.[19]

doi: 10.1111/j.1749-6632.2012.06804.x
Ann. N.Y. Acad. Sci. 1275 (2012) 23–28 © 2012 New York Academy of Sciences.

MTX is an analog of folic acid and is an antimetabolite and a potent inhibitor of dihydrofolate reductase,[20] which subsequently inhibits *de novo* purine and pyrimidine synthesis. It originated in the 1940s when Dr. Sidney Farber at Children's Hospital Boston was testing the effects of folic acid on acute leukemic children. MTX gained U.S. Food and Drug Administration approval as an oncology drug in 1953. Once intracellular, MTX is bioactivated to the polyglutamated form of MTX ($MTXglu_n$) by folylpolyglutamyl synthase (FPGS), which promotes cellular retention and inhibition of several enzymes.[21] No or low glutamation leads to the efflux of MTX by the ATP-binding cassette (ABC) family of transporters. *FPGS* and *ABCG2* are of particular interest as folate deprivation has been associated with increased expression of *FPGS* and decreased expression of *ABCG2*,[22] suggesting a cellular response to low folate with an increase in polyglutamation and decrease in folate export to promote retention of folate within the cell. Additionally, upregulation of *ABCG2* protein expression has been associated with MTX resistance in cancer cells.[23] Therefore, allelic variation in these genes resulting in increased or decreased activity may be associated with either increased or decreased $MTXglu_n$. This entire process is also likely dependent upon the folate status of the patient, reflected by the polyglutamation of folate itself, and the relative concentrations of the two groups of mutually antagonistic compounds.

As serum MTX concentrations have been notoriously unreliably associated with MTX clinical outcomes,[24–26] the search for more stable biomarkers of disease response to MTX has been ongoing. An association between RBC $MTXglu_n$ and effectiveness of MTX in RA has been reported.[27,28] Higher levels of "long chain $MTXglu_n$" (defined as $MTXglu_3$ or greater) were associated with improved effectiveness of MTX in RA. Since RBC folate concentrations are established during erythropoiesis and represent the average folate status over the preceding 120 days,[29] by extension, MTX concentrations in RBCs are a surrogate biomarker of average drug exposure over a similar period of time. Furthermore, MTX polyglutamates in RBCs are considered to be representative of intracellular MTX levels in target tissues, are more stable than serum levels of MTX, and may potentially predict response to the drug.[27,28,30,31]

Methods

We have designed a randomized, double-blinded, controlled trial of MTX versus placebo in MG patients who are on steroids. Patients aged 18 years or older with MGFA grade is 2, 3, or 4 are enrolled in this study. They should have an elevated acetylcholine receptor antibody (AChR-Ab) titer and be on a stable prednisone dose of at least 10 mg/day or the equivalent, with alternate day dosing for 30 days before the screening visit. They should not have thymoma, tumor, infection, or interstitial lung disease. Those excluded from this study are patients who had a thymectomy in the previous three months, those that have been on immunosuppressive therapy within the last 60 days, those using daily nonsteroidal anti-inflammatory drugs, those having renal or hepatic insufficiency or elevated liver enzymes, and those with prior use of MTX for MG or any other condition within the prior two years. Potential patients signed informed consent and underwent baseline laboratory testing. Subjects are randomly assigned with equal allocation to the two treatment arms (MTX or placebo) stratified by baseline prednisone dose (≥ 30 mg day or < 30 mg day, or the equivalent for every other day dosing) based on the randomization plan developed by the Department of Biostatistics at the University of Kansas Medical Center. All subjects had a baseline evaluation, including a complete history, neurological examination, quantitative MG score (QMG), MG activities of daily living (MG-ADL) score, MG composite score, and MG quality of life-15 (MGQOL-15). This is followed by a similar evaluation every four weeks for 12 months. In addition, adverse events and changes in a patient's history and medications are documented at each follow-up visit. Blood is drawn at visit 12 for MTX polyglutamate estimation in RBC. Patients receive MTX 10 mg weekly or placebo, and if there are no clinical or laboratory side effects, the dose is increased to 15 mg weekly at two weeks, and increased to 20 mg weekly at five weeks. All participants also receive folic acid to be taken daily to prevent stomatitis. Prednisone tapering is started at the month 3 visit and monthly thereafter, according to a predetermined protocol based on the MG symptoms. The dose is increased if symptoms worsen.

Outcome measures and statistical analysis

The primary measure of efficacy is the nine-month prednisone area (months 3–12) under the time dose curve (AUC),[32] which measures the total prednisone doses of each patient for nine months. A reduction of prednisone AUC demonstrates that patients improved on clinical grounds so that the prednisone dose could be decreased per protocol. Secondary outcome measures are the change of Quantitative Myasthenia Gravis Score (QMG) from baseline. We will also analyze the 12-month changes in the MG-ADL, MG QOL-15, MMT scores, composite MG score, reduction in prednisone side effects, prednisone dose change from the baseline visit to visit 15, prednisone dose AUC months 7–12, the number of patients achieving minimal manifestations or pharmacological remission, time to worsening of MG symptoms, number of worsening episodes, number of plasmapheresis patients receive from day 90 to day 360, the number of treatment failures in each group, prednisone dose at each visit, and the AUC prednisone dose only for patients who did not receive any plasmapheresis during the study. At the end of the study, a stratified log-rank test will be used to compare the treatment groups with regard to the time (from randomization) until treatment failure. Fisher's exact test will be used with regard to the number of patients achieving minimal manifestations or pharmacological remission and the numbers of worsening episodes. All the other continuous secondary outcome measures will be analyzed using the two sample *t* test. Data will be analyzed in an intent-to-treat fashion. This will be accomplished as an analysis of covariance examining the change from initial to final value as the outcome result and the initial value as a covariate.

Results

Fifty-six subjects have been screened to date with 50 enrolled and 6 screen failures. Out of the 50 patients enrolled, 21 patients have completed the study, 1 patient died from a non-study medication–related event, and 5 patients withdrew, owing to a new diagnosis of Parkinson disease, ALT elevation, myalgia, transportation problems, and poor tolerability, respectively. A total of 23 patients are currently active in the study.

Discussion

Drugs such as azathioprine,[33,34] cyclophosphamide,[35] cyclosporine,[36,37] mycophenolate mofetil,[1–4] and intravenous immunoglobulin (IVIg)[38,39] have been studied with varying degrees of success in MG. Like steroids, all have undesirable side effects, including hypertension, renal insufficiency, and hirsutism associated with cyclosporine, cystitis, myelosuppression, and mutagenicity with cyclophosphamide, and systemic hypersensitivity, hepatotoxicity, and myelosuppression with azathioprine.[40] Plasma exchange has been successfully used to lower the titer of AChR-Abs, with clinical improvement in some patients.[41] However, because of the technical difficulties and medical morbidity associated with chronic plasma exchange, it is a therapy that is now usually reserved for respiratory crisis. Recently two multicenter-controlled trials of mycophenolate mofetil showed no benefit in MG.[1–4] These disappointing findings have prompted interest in looking for other immunosuppressive drugs that are currently available and have led to our interest in MTX for MG. There have been few small studies that showed the efficacy of MTX in MG.[16–18] However, our study is the first randomized double-blind placebo controlled trial of methotrexate.

The three positive MG studies (i.e., cyclosporine and IVIg), where QMG was used as the primary endpoint, were short, 4- to 12-weeks.[36–38] In the positive azathioprine study, the benefit of the drug was not seen until month 12 using the prednisone dose as the primary end point.[34] One of the post hoc criticisms of the mycophenolate study was that it was only a three-month trial. Therefore, for this MTX trial we have planned a 12-month trial. In the azathioprine trial in MG, the beneficial effects of azathioprine were not seen for 12 months,[34] so we believe that new trials need to be at least this long.

The MTX polyglutamates in RBC will also be estimated in this study that has not been done previously in other MG MTX studies. MTX polyglutamates in RBCs are considered to be representative of intracellular MTX levels in target tissues, are more stable than serum levels of MTX, and may potentially predict response to the drug.[27,28,30,31]

The QMG was initially suggested as the best objective measure for use in MG clinical trials.[42]

This score was used by Tindall *et al.* in double-blind, randomized, placebo-controlled studies of cyclosporine in myasthenia gravis.[36,37] Tindall found that an improvement of 4 points in QMG was associated with a sustained clinical change. This score was used in the completed MG trials of mycophenolate mofetil[1–4] and IVIg.[38,39] In the recently completed study of IVIg in MG, the patients receiving IVIg improved by 2.5 units, an additional 1.6 units compared to placebo. However, we are not using the QMG as the primary efficacy measure in this study because we are concerned that we may not observe a significant difference between these two groups in relation to QMG change even if MTX is effective. This is due to the fact that both groups are on prednisone, and the prednisone dose of each patient may be increased or decreased depending on the patient's condition. Because this is a long (12-month) study, it is very possible that increasing prednisone dose could be necessary. A dose change may subsequently affect the patient's QMG. Therefore, the prednisone dosing may confound the treatment effect with respect to the QMG. It is possible that patients in both groups will ultimately improve so that we cannot determine a difference with the QMG. For this reason, the QMG will be used as a secondary rather than the primary end point.

The primary measure of efficacy in our study will be the nine-month prednisone AUC (months 3–12), which measures the total prednisone doses of each patient in nine months. A reduction of prednisone AUC demonstrates that patients improved on clinical grounds so that the prednisone dose could be decreased. If the patients receiving MTX have a smaller prednisone AUC compared to the placebo patients, this will have demonstrated the efficacy of MTX. Our biostatisticians will determine if both placebo and MTX groups are equivalent for subject weight as part of the analysis. A daily prednisone drug diary is maintained by patients, and this information will be used to calculate the AUC measurements. The two-sample *t* test will be used to test the difference between the mean AUCs of the two treatment groups under the assumption that the distribution of AUC is approximately normal. The normality assumption was satisfactorily tested in a comparable study,[34] which used the median maintenance prednisolone dose as the primary measure to test the efficacy of azathioprine plus prednisone versus prednisone plus placebo. Without prior informa-tion about prednisone AUC with MTX, we used information from the Palace study for the sample size consideration because these two studies have a similar design. Data derived from the Palace study showed a mean AUC that is nearly three times its standard deviation in the prednisone plus placebo group, and the mean/SD value based on the pooled data from both groups is about 2. To be more conservative, we assume a mean/SD ratio of 2.5 for the placebo group. Twenty patients in each study arm provides 0.8 power of detecting a 0.784 effect size (mean change/SD), which is equivalent to a 31.4% reduction in total prednisone doses in nine months for the MTX group over the placebo group. Assuming a drop-out rate of 20%, anticipated enrollment is a total of 50 participants (25 patients in the treatment group and 25 patients in the placebo group).

Similar to other previous MG studies, the enrollment has been a challenge and a slow process. However, we anticipate complete enrollment by December 2012 and clinical follow-up for another 12 months. We started with six sites initially, and due to challenges with enrollment, other sites were included. Presently there are 18 U.S. sites and two Canadian sites participating in this study.

Acknowledgments

This study was funded by Food and Drug Administration Orphan Products Division RO1 FD 003538. Additional funding was provided in part by Grants UL1 RR 033179 (which is now UL1 TR 000001) from the University of Kansas Medical Center Clinical and Translational Science Awards (CTSA). Muscle Study Group: University of Kansas Medical Center: R.J.B., MD (PI); M.P., MD (co-PI); M.D., MD; L.H. (project manager); University of Texas Southwestern Medical Center: Sharon Nations, MD (PI); University of Texas Health Science Center San Antonio: Carlayne Jackson, MD (PI); University of Virginia: Ted Burns (PI); University of Miami: Michael Benatar, MD (PI); Ohio State University: Bakri Elsheikh (PI); University of California, Irvine: A.W., MD (PI); University of San Francisco–Fresno (J.R., MD (PI); Indiana University: R.P., MD (PI); University of North Carolina: J. Howard, MD (PI); Massachusetts General Hospital: David Walk, MD (PI); California Pacific Medical Center: Jonathan Katz, MD (PI); University of Iowa Hospitals and Clinics: Andrea Swenson, MD (PI); Nerve and Muscle Center in Texas: Aziz Shaibani,

MD (PI); The Methodist Hospital System: Ericka Simpson, MD (PI); Penn State Hershey: Matthew Wicklund, MD (PI); Phoenix Neurological Center: David Saperstein (PI); University of Florida-Jacksonville: Michael Pulley, MD (PI); University of Toronto: Vera Bril, MD (PI); McGill University: Angela Genge, MD (PI); and Children's Mercy Hospital and Clinics (for polyglutamation assays), Mara Becker, MD. Muscle Study Group (MSG) Steering Committee: Annabel Wang, MD, T.B., MD; R.J.B., MD; M.P., MD; L.H. and J. (Wendy) H., PhD. Safety Monitoring Committee: Kevin Latinis, MD (chair); Anthony Amato, MD; Erik Ensrud, MD; and Jonathan Goldstein, MD.

Conflicts of interest

The authors declare no conflicts of interest.

References

1. Sanders, D., M. McDermott, C. Thornton, *et al.* 2007. A trial of mycophenolate mofetil (MMF) with prednisone as initial immunotherapy in myasthenia gravis (MG) [abstract]. *Neurology* **62**(Suppl 1)**:** 107.
2. Sanders, D.B., I.K. Hart, R. Mantegazza, *et al.* 2008. An international, phase III, randomized trial of mycophenolate mofetil in myasthenia gravis. *Neurology* **71**(6): 400–406.
3. Sanders, D. & Z. Siddiqi. 2008. Lessons from two trials of mycophenolate mofetil in myasthenia gravis. *Ann. N.Y. Acad. Sci.* **1132**: 249–253.
4. The Muscle Study Group. 2008. A trial of mycophenolate mofetil with prednisone as initial immunotherapy in myasthenia gravis. *Neurology* **71**: 394–399.
5. Furst, D.F. & J.M. Kremer. 1988. Methotrexate in rheumatoid arthritis. *Arthritis Rheum.* **31**: 305–314.
6. Hirata, S., T. Matsubara, R. Saura, *et al.* 1989. Inhibition of in vitro vascular endothelial cell proliferation and in vivo neovascularization by low-dose methotrexate. *Arthritis Rheum.* **3**: 1065–1073.
7. Kremer, J.M. & J.K. Lee. 1988. A long term prospective study of the use of methotrexate in rheumatoid arthritis. Update after a mean of fifty-three months. *Arthritis Rheum.* **31**: 577–584.
8. Lange, F., E. Bajtner, C. Rintisch, *et al.* 2005. Methotrexate ameliorates T cell dependent autoimmune arthritis and encephalomyelitis but not antibody induced or fibroblast induced arthritis. *Ann. Rheum. Dis.* **64**: 599–605.
9. Nakajima, A., M. Hakoda, H. Yamanaka, *et al.* 1996. Divergent effects of methotrexate on the clonal growth of T and B lymphocytes and synovial adherent cells from patients with rheumatoid arthritis. *Ann. Rheum. Dis.* **55**: 237–42.
10. Rau, R., G. Herborn, T. Karger & D. Werdier. 1991. Retardation of radiologic progression in rheumatoid arthritis with methotrexate therapy. *Arthritis Rheum.* **34**: 1236–1244.
11. Segal, R., E. Mozes, M. Yaron & B. Tartakovsky. 1989. The effects of methotrexate on the production and activity of interleukin-1. *Arthritis Rheum.* **32**: 370–7.
12. Weinblatt, M.E., B.N. Weissman, D.E. Holdsworth, *et al.* 1992. Long-term prospective study of methotrexate in the treatment of rheumatoid arthritis. 84-month update. *Arthritis Rheum.* **35**: 129–137.
13. Currier, R.D., A.F. Haerer & E.F. Meydrech. 1993. Low dose oral methotrexate treatment of multiple sclerosis: a pilot study. *J. Neurol. Neurosurg. Psych.* **56**: 1217–18.
14. Goodkin, D.E., R.A. Rudick, S. VanderBrug Medendorp, *et al.* 1995. Low dose (7.5 mg) oral methotrexate reduces the rate of progression in chronic progressive multiple sclerosis. *Ann. Neurol.* **37**: 30–40.
15. Goodkin, D.E., R.A. Rudick, S. VanderBrug Medendorp, *et al.* 1996. Low-dose oral methotrexate in chronic progressive multiple sclerosis: analyses of serial MRIs. *Neurology* **47**: 1153–1157.
16. Abdou, A.M. 2007. Methotrexate for treatment of myasthenia gravis. *Neurology* **62**(Suppl 1): 300–301.
17. Hartmann, J. & M.H. Rivner. 2009. Methotrexate in myasthenia gravis. *Clin. Neurophysiol.* 120: e123–e124
18. Heckmann, J.M., A. Rawoot, K. Bateman, *et al.* 2011. A single-blinded trial of methotrexate versus azathioprine as steroid-sparing agents in generalized myasthenia gravis. *BMC Neurol.* **11**: 97.
19. Raja, F.M., M.M. Dimachkie, A.L. McVey, *et al.* 2009. Methotrexate in the treatment of myasthenia gravis. *Neurology* 72(Suppl 3): A54.
20. Calabresi, P. & B. Chabner. 1990. Antineoplastic agents. In *The Pharmalogical Basis of Therapeutics.* 8th ed. A. Gilman, T. Rall, A. Nies & P. Taylor, Eds.: 1209–1263. Pergamon. New York.
21. Chabner, B.A., C.J. Allegra, G.A. Curt, *et al.* 1985. Polyglutamation of Methotrexate. Is Methotrexate a pro drug? *J. Clin. Invest.* **76**: 907–912.
22. Ifergan, I., A. Shafran, G. Jansen, *et al.* 2004. Folate deprivation results in the loss of breast cancer resistance protein (BCRP/ABCG2) expression. A role for BCRP in cellular folate homeostasis. *J. Biol. Chem.* **279**: 25527.
23. Volker, L. & E. Schneider. 2003. Wild type breast cancer resistance protein (BCRP/ABCG2) is a methotrexate polyglutamate transporter. *Cancer Res.* **63**: 5538–5543.
24. Lafforgue, P., S. Monjanel-Mouterde, A. Durand, *et al.* 1995. Lack of correlation between pharamkokinetics and efficacy of low dose methotrexate in patients with rheumatoid arthritis. *J. Rheum.* **22**: 844–849.
25. Ravelli, A., G. Di Fuccia, M. Molinaro, *et al.* 1993. Plasma levels after oral methotrexate in children with juvenile rheumatoid arthritis. *J. Rheum.* **20**: 1573–1577.
26. Wallace, C.A., W.A. Bleyer, D.D. Sherry, *et al.* 1989. Toxicity and serum levels of methotrexate in children with juvenile rheumatoid arthritis. *Arthritis Rheum.* **32**: 677–681.
27. Dervieux, T., J. Kremer, D. Orentas Lein, *et al.* 2004. Contribution of common polymorphisms in reduced folate carrier and γ-glutamylhydrolase to Methotrexate polyglutamate levels in patients with rheumatoid arthritis. *Pharmacogenetics* **14**: 733–739.

28. Derivieux, T., D. Furst, D. Orentas Lein, *et al.* 2005. Pharmacogenetic and metabolite measurements are associated with clinical status in patients with rheumatoid arthritis treated with Methotrexate: results of a multicentered cross sectional observational study. *Ann. Rheum. Dis.* **64:** 1180–1185.

29. Herbert, V. 1987. Making sense of laboratory tests of folate status: folate requirements to sustain normality. *Am. J. Hematol.* **26:** 199–207.

30. Dalrymple, J.M., L.K. Stamp, J.L. O'Donnell, *et al.* 2008. Pharmacokinetics of oral methotrexate in patients with rheumatoid arthritis. *Arthritis Rheum.* **58:** 3299–3308.

31. Stamp, L.K., J.L. O'Donnell, P.T. Chapman, *et al.* 2009. Determinants of red blood cell methotrexate polyglutamate concentrations in rheumatoid arthritis patients receiving long-term methotrexate treatment. *Arthritis Rheum.* **60:** 2248–2256.

32. Benatar, M., D.B. Sanders, T.M. Burns, *et al.* 2012. Recommendations for myasthenia gravis clinical trials. *Muscle Nerve* **45:** 909–917.

33. Mertens, H.G., P. Hertel, P. Reuther & K. Ricker. 1981. Effect of immunosuppressive drugs (azathioprine). *Ann. N.Y. Acad. Sci.* **377:** 691–699.

34. Palace, J., J. Newsom-Davis & B. Lecky. 1998. A randomized double-blind trial of prednisolone alone or with azathioprine in myasthenia gravis. *Neurology* **50:** 1778–1783.

35. Drachman, D.B., R.J. Jones & R.A. Brodsky. 2003. Treatment of refractory myasthenia: "Rebooting" with high-dose cyclophosphamide. *Ann. Neurol.* **53:** 29–34.

36. Tindall R.S.A., J.A. Rollins, J.T. Phillips, *et al.* 1987. Preliminary results of a double-blind, randomized, placebo-controlled trial of cyclosporine in myasthenia gravis. *N. Engl. J. Med.* **316:** 719–724.

37. Tindall, R.S.A., J.T. Phillips, J.A. Rollins, *et al.* 1992. A clinical therapeutic trial of cyclosporine in myasthenia gravis. *Ann. N.Y. Acad. Sci.* **681:** 539–551.

38. Zinman, L., E. Ng & V. Bril. 2007. IV immunoglobulin in patients with myasthenia gravis: a randomized controlled trial. *Neurology* **68:** 837–841.

39. Wolfe, G.I., R.J. Barohn, B.M. Foster, *et al.* 2002. Randomized, controlled trial of intravenous immunoglobulin in myasthenia gravis. *Muscle Nerve* **26:** 549–552.

40. Kissel, J.T., R.j. Levy, J.R. Mendell & R.C. Griggs. 1986. Azathioprine toxicity in neuromuscular disease. *Neurology* **36:** 35–39.

41. Dau, P.C., J.M. Lindstrom, C.K. Cassel, *et al.* 1977. Plasmaphereses and immunosuppressive drug therapy in myasthenia gravis. *N. Engl. J. Med.* **297:** 1134–1140.

42. Jaretzski, A., III, R.J. Barohn, R.M. Ernstoff, *et al.* 2000. Myasthenia gravis: recommendations for clinical research standards. *Ann. Thorac. Surg.* **70:** 327–334.

Ann. N.Y. Acad. Sci. ISSN 0077-8923

Identification of *DPAGT1* as a new gene in which mutations cause a congenital myasthenic syndrome

Katsiaryna Belaya,[1] Sarah Finlayson,[1,2] Judith Cossins,[1] Wei Wei Liu,[1] Susan Maxwell,[1] Jacqueline Palace,[2] and David Beeson[1]

[1]Neurosciences Group, Nuffield Department of Clinical Neurosciences, Weatherall Institute of Molecular Medicine, University of Oxford, Oxford, United Kingdom. [2]Nuffield Department of Clinical Neurosciences, John Radcliffe Hospital, Oxford, United Kingdom

Address for correspondence: Dr. Katsiaryna Belaya, Weatherall Institute of Molecular Medicine, University of Oxford, Oxford, OX3 9DS, UK. katsiaryna.belaya@dpag.ox.ac.uk

Congenital myasthenic syndromes (CMS) are a group of inherited disorders that arise from impaired signal transmission at the neuromuscular synapse. They are characterized by fatigable muscle weakness. This is a heterogenous group of disorders with 15 different genes implicated in the development of the disease. Using whole-exome sequencing we identified *DPAGT1* as a new gene associated with CMS. DPAGT1 catalyses the first step of *N*-linked protein glycosylation. *DPAGT1* patients are characterized by weakness of limb muscles, response to treatment with cholinesterase inhibitors, and the presence of tubular aggregates on muscle biopsy. We showed that *DPAGT1* is required for glycosylation of acetylcholine receptor (AChR) subunits and efficient export of AChR to the cell surface. We suggest that the primary pathogenic mechanism of *DPAGT1*-associated CMS is reduced levels of AChRs at the endplate region. This finding demonstrates that impairment of the *N*-linked glycosylation pathway can lead to the development of CMS.

Keywords: AChR; congenital myasthenic syndrome; *DPAGT1*; glycosylation; neuromuscular junction

Identification of *DPAGT1* as a new gene associated with congenital myasthenic syndrome

Congenital myasthenic syndromes (CMS) are hereditary disorders of neuromuscular transmission.[1,2] They are characterized by fatigable muscle weakness that often affects ocular, bulbar, limb, or respiratory muscles. The onset of the disease is usually within infancy or early childhood, but some cases with late onset have been described. The severity of disease varies greatly from mild muscular weakness throughout life to death in early childhood.

To date, mutations in 15 different genes have been implicated in the development of CMS.[1,2] These genes encode the presynaptic protein (CHAT), synaptic components (COLQ, AGRN, LAMB2), and postsynaptic proteins (CHRNA1, CHRNB1, CHRNG, CHRND, CHRNE, RAPSN, MUSK, DOK7, GFPT1, PLEC, SCN4A). For the majority

of these proteins, their function at the neuromuscular junction has been well established. Some proteins are required for the transmission of the signal from neuron to the muscle, while others are needed for the establishment and maintenance of the synapse structure. However, for some of these proteins, it still remains unclear what their role at the neuromuscular junction (NMJ) is and how mutations in these genes can lead to the development of CMS. For example, *GFPT1* has recently been implicated in the development of CMS.[3] *GFPT1* encodes glutamine-fructose-6-phosphate transaminase 1. This is an enzyme that catalyzes the first and rate-limiting step of the hexosamine pathway. The end product of the hexosamine pathway is uridine diphospho-*N*-acetylglucosamine (UDP-GlcNAc)—a nucleotide sugar donor that serves as a substrate for *N*-linked and *O*-linked protein glycosylation, as well as for glycosylation of lipids and proteoglycans. *GFPT1* is ubiquitously expressed and it is not clear how mutations in such an essential gene

doi: 10.1111/j.1749-6632.2012.06790.x

Table 1. *DPAGT1* mutations found in CMS patients

	Mutation, DNA	Mutation, protein
Case 1	c.[324G>C]; [349G>A]	p.[Met108Ile]; [Val117Ile]
Case 2	c.[349G>A]; [699dup]	p.[Val117Ile]; [Thr234Hisfs*116]
Case 3	c.[478G>A(;)574G>A]	p.[Gly160Ser(;)Gly192Ser]
Cases 4 and 5	c.[358C>A]; [791T>G]	p.[Leu120Met]; [Val264Gly]

can specifically lead to a neuromuscular phenotype, without having a more generalized effect.

CMS cases with mutations in the *GFPT1* gene have clinical features that can help distinguish them from the majority of CMS patients.[4] They are characterized by a predominantly limb-girdle pattern of muscle weakness, later onset of the disease, presence of tubular aggregates on muscle biopsies, and response to treatment with cholinesterase inhibitors.

There is a subset of CMS patients with symptoms similar to *GFPT1* patients, but without mutations in *GFPT1*. We have performed whole-exome capture and next-generation sequencing from two of such patients and identified a new gene—*DPAGT1*—in which mutations cause CMS.[5] Screening of a further cohort of CMS patients with varying clinical features allowed us to identify three more patients with mutations in this gene, bringing the total number of patients with *DPAGT1*-associated CMS to five (Table 1). All mutations found in these patients lie in conserved regions of the protein and are likely to be important for protein function (Fig. 1). All five patients have clinical symptoms characteristic of CMS: a decrement on 3-Hz repetitive nerve stimulation and jitter and blocking on single fiber EMG. The most severely affected muscle groups are proximal and distal limb muscles, while the effect on facial, ocular, bulbar, and respiratory muscles is minimal. The age of onset is during childhood, rather than birth or infancy. Similar to *GFPT1* patients, analyzed *DPAGT1* patients have tubular aggregates present on their muscle biopsies. Patients showed a good response to treatment with pyridostigmine (a cholinesterase inhibitor), and two benefited from taking 3,4-diaminopyridine (a drug that increases acetylcholine release from the nerve terminal). Thus, *DPAGT1* patients have clinical features that show similarities to *GFPT1* CMS but should help distinguish them from the rest of CMS patients.

DPAGT1 encodes dolichyl-phosphate (UDP-*N*-acetylglucosamine) *N*-acetylglucosaminephosphotransferase 1 (EC number 2.7.8.15), which catalyses the first committed step of *N*-linked protein glycosylation.[6] *N*-linked protein glycosylation is an essential form of posttranslational protein modification. The pathway of *N*-linked glycosylation is conserved in all eukaryotes.[7,8] It is a multistep process that involves coordinated functioning of multiple proteins (Fig. 2). It starts with the assembly of the core glycan ($Glc_3Man_9GlcNAc_2$) on the lipid dolichol. The assembly of the core glycan happens in the endoplasmic reticulum (ER) and is carried out by a series of membrane bound enzymes. These enzymes sequentially add monosaccharides to the lipid dolichol. Once the core glycan is assembled, it is transferred from the lipid dolichol onto the asparagine residues of nascent proteins. The core glycan can then undergo a series of trimming and extension events that happen in the ER and Golgi and result in the formation of a complex carbohydrate structure found on mature proteins.

Glycosylation of proteins serves many important biological functions including protein folding and stability, intracellular targeting, cell signaling, intercellular recognition, and others.[7,9] Thus, it is not surprising that disruption of the glycosylation pathway leads to the development of serious multisystem disorders. Mutations in different proteins involved in glycan biosynthesis have been described, and the resulting conditions are generally called congenital disorders of glycosylation (CDG). The exact subtype of CDG depends on which particular gene has been disrupted. For example, mutations in PMM2 gene lead to the development of PMM2-CDG (or CDG1A), mutations in the MPI gene will lead to the development of MPI-CDG (or CDG1B), and so on. Most of CDGs are multisystem diseases that simultaneously affect various organs. Manifestations include developmental delay, mental retardation,

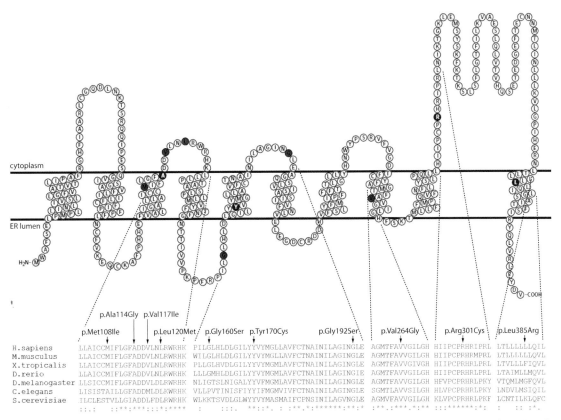

Figure 1. Predicted membrane topology of the DPAGT1 protein. Residues that are mutated in CMS patients are shown in red. Residues that are mutated in CDG1J patients are shown in blue. Transmembrane structure of the protein was visualized using TEXtopo.[29] Multiple sequence alignment was performed using ClustalW.[30]

various neuromuscular defects, hormonal abnormalities, and dysmorphic features.[9] However, there are notable exceptions of patients who present with a more organ-restricted phenotype. For example, in CDG1B patients with mutations in MPI (mannose phosphate isomerase) neurological symptoms are usually absent and the most affected organs are the gastrointestinal tract and liver.[10] On the other hand, the symptoms of CDG1O patients with mutations in DPM3 (dolichyl-phosphate mannosyltransferase polypeptide 3) can be limited to a muscular dystrophy phenotype.[11]

DPAGT1 transfers the first sugar—GlcNAc—from the UDP-GlcNAc onto the lipid dolichol.[6] Notably, UDP-GlcNAc is an end product of the hexosamine pathway—the pathway containing GFPT1. Thus, both GFPT1 and DPAGT1 are involved in the same cellular process. The human DPAGT1 is 408 amino acids long and is predicted to span the ER membrane ten times[12] (Fig. 1). DPAGT1

is essential for survival, as *Dpagt1* knockout mice die shortly after implantation.[13] Four patients with mutations in *DPAGT1* have been previously described and all have been classified as CDG1J patients.[14–16] Similar to CMS patients, mutations identified in CDG1J patients disrupt conserved amino acids (Fig. 1). All four patients had severe clinical phenotypes that affect multiple organ systems. The first reported patient had delayed development, severe hypotonia, microcephaly, medically intractable seizures, and mental retardation.[15] The second and third patients were siblings from a consanguineous family and had delayed development, hypotonia, intractable seizures, and microcephaly, and both died within the first year of life.[16] The final patient had severe fetal hypokinesia, moderate multiple contractures, camptodactyly, hypotonia with no spontaneous movement, and died at 1.5 months of age.[14] Interestingly, all four patients had severe hypotonia, suggesting that the

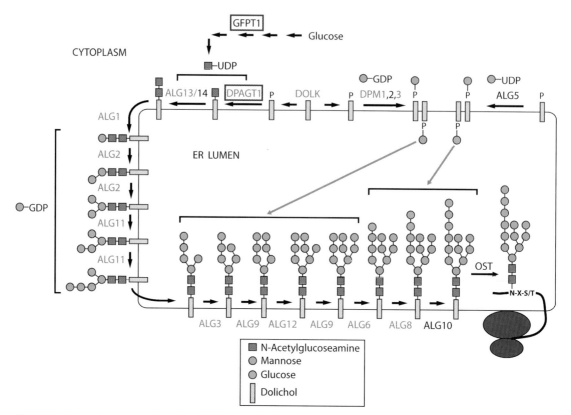

Figure 2. Schematic representation of the *N*-linked protein glycosylation pathway. *N*-linked protein glycosylation takes place in the ER. It starts with the assembly of the core glycan on the lipid dolichol. Different saccharides are added to the lipid sequentially by different enzymes. The first stage of oligosaccharide assembly takes place on the cytoplasmic face of the ER, where a series of glycosyltransferases uses a cytoplasmic pool of soluble nucleotide sugar donors as substrates for dolichol glycosylation. These nucleotide-monosaccharides are synthesized by multiple cytosolic enzymes, one of which is GFPT1 (involved in the synthesis of UDP-GlcNAc). The first sugar—*N*-acetylglucoseamine (GlcNAc)—is added to dolichol by the enzyme DPAGT1. The second GlcNAc is transferred by the Alg13/Alg14 complex, where Alg13 is a catalytic subunit and Alg14 is an anchoring subunit that targets Alg13 to the ER membrane. Addition of the first mannose is carried out by Alg1, while Alg2 and Alg11 sequentially add four more mannose residues. Next, the resulting Dol-P-P-GlcNAc$_2$Man$_5$ intermediate is flipped so that the oligosaccharide is facing inside the ER lumen. This step is carried out by an as yet unknown mechanism. Addition of subsequent sugar moieties is carried out inside the ER lumen. Here, the monosaccharide donor substrates are dolichyl-phosphate–linked monosaccharides Dol-P-mannose and Dol-P-glucose, which are synthesized on the cytoplasmic face of the ER by Dpm1/2/3 and Alg5 enzymes, respectively. Extension of Dol-P-oligosaccharide is carried out by Alg3, Alg9, and Alg12, which add four mannose residues. The final three glucose residues are added by Alg6, Alg8, and Alg10, completing the assembly of the core glycan. The core glycan is then transferred to asparagine residues of nascent proteins by the multimeric oligosaccharyl transferase complex (OST). The core glycan can then be modified inside the ER and Golgi to yield the final complex saccharide structure found on the mature proteins. Mutations in many of the enzymes of the *N*-linked protein glycosylation pathway have been associated with diseases. In this figure, genes in which mutations are known to lead to the development of CDG disorders are shown in blue. Genes in which mutations cause development of CMS are enclosed in red boxes.

neuromuscular function in these patients was seriously compromised.

Thus, disruption of normal neuromuscular function is a feature reported for both CDG1J and CMS patients. In terms of other characteristics, the patients with *DPAGT1*-associated CMS differ from CDG1J patients, since they do not display the non-

muscle symptoms typical of CDG1J. It is as yet unclear why mutations in the same gene can lead to a different clinical presentation. It is possible that the mutations in the CMS patients are less damaging than the mutations found in CDG1J patients, so that DPAGT1 retains sufficient activity in the majority of tissues. The neuromuscular junction might be especially sensitive to the disruption of *DPAGT1*, so that even a minor reduction in DPAGT1 activity might be sufficient to cause a phenotype. In the future, it will be interesting to measure catalytic activity of different *DPAGT1* mutants and compare mutations leading to the development of CMS to those leading to the development of CDG1J. These experiments should help elucidate how different mutations in the same gene can lead to the development of different disorders.

The role of *DPAGT1* at the neuromuscular junction

Since *DPAGT1* is required for *N*-linked protein glycosylation, it is likely that disruption of this gene leads to a defect in glycosylation of one or several NMJ components. It is known that multiple components of NMJ are glycosylated. Notable examples include the subunits of the AChR receptor, Agrin and Musk (both of which are essential for clustering of AChR receptors at the endplate region), and laminin.[17]

To establish the effect that mutations in *DPAGT1* have on the structure of NMJ, we analyzed muscle biopsies from patients with *DPAGT1* mutations. The endplates from these patients displayed two notable abnormalities.[5] First, the amount of postsynaptic folding present at the endplate region was reduced fivefold compared to control muscles. The reduction in postsynaptic folds is likely to coincide with a decrease in the number of available voltage-gated sodium channels that are concentrated in the depths of the postsynaptic folds. This will increase the threshold depolarization required for triggering the action potential.[18,19] Second, the amount of acetylcholine receptor present at the endplate of *DPAGT1* patients was decreased. Reduced levels of AChR decrease the sensitivity of the postsynaptic membrane to the neurotransmitter acetylcholine. Taken together, these two defects reduce the safety factor for neuromuscular transmission and are sufficient to explain the muscle weakness observed in the patients. Notably, similar abnormalities of the NMJ ultrastructure are characteristically observed in AChR deficiency patients, where the amount of AChR that is present at the NMJ is significantly reduced.[20–22] Both AChR deficiency patients and *DPAGT1* CMS patients benefit from treatment with cholinesterase inhibitors.[2,5] In combination, these results indicate that for patients with mutations in *DPAGT1*, the likely primary cause of the weakness is a reduction of AChR at the endplate region.

Adult AChR is a pentameric receptor consisting of two alpha, one beta, one delta, and one epsilon subunits. The pentamer is assembled in the ER.[23] All subunits of the AChR undergo *N*-linked glycosylation in the ER, which is required for appropriate assembly of the pentamer and for the insertion of the AChR into the plasma membrane.[24–26] It is possible that disruption of DPAGT1 function leads to abnormal glycosylation of AChR subunits and therefore prevents insertion of the receptor into the plasma membrane.

Using the DPAGT1-specific inhibitor tunicamycin, we showed that DPAGT1 is indeed required for glycosylation of AChR subunits.[5] Addition of tunicamycin to cells transfected with AChR subunits led to a loss in subunit glycosylation, while overexpression of wild-type *DPAGT1* in these cells rescued the inhibition with tunicamycin. In accordance, treatment of cells with tunicamycin resulted in a fivefold reduction in the amount of AChR inserted into the plasma membrane compared to non-treated cells. At the same time, overexpression of wild-type DPAGT1 protein in these cells restored the normal levels of AChR inserted into the plasma membrane. These results demonstrate that DPAGT1 is required for glycosylation of AChR subunits and for export of AChR to the cell surface. This proposed pathogenic mechanism is in keeping with the phenotype observed in the patient muscle biopsies, where the levels of AChR in the endplate region are reduced.

We thus propose that the primary defect in *DPAGT1* CMS patients is loss of AChR from the NMJ region due to deficient glycosylation of AChR subunits. It is likely that the same mechanism explains the neuromuscular weakness observed in *GFPT1*-associated CMS. It is not yet clear whether glycosylation of other NMJ proteins is affected in *DPAGT1* patients, and what effect they might have on the development of the disease.

Tubular aggregates

An interesting feature common to both *DPAGT1* and *GFPT1* CMS patients is the presence of tubular aggregates on muscle biopsy. To date all analyzed *DPAGT1* patients and the majority of *GFPT1* patients have this feature. The exact nature of tubular aggregates is as yet unknown. They are usually characterized as structures composed of membranes and protein, and they are believed to arise from the membranes of sarcoplasmic reticulum, and are thought to be filled with unfolded or misfolded protein.[27,28] It is possible that in CMS patients with mutations in *DPAGT1* and *GFPT1* genes, several cellular proteins become abnormally glycosylated, fail to be properly folded, and accumulate in the sarcoplasmic reticulum, leading to the formation of tubular aggregates. It will be of interest to determine the molecular composition of tubular aggregates in the muscles from these CMS patients.

Conclusions and future perspectives

Our recent identification of *DPAGT1* as a novel gene in which mutations cause CMS, together with the recently published papers on *GFPT1*-associated CMS, highlight a new pathway leading to the development of NMJ disorders. Both *DPAGT1* and *GFPT1* are involved in protein glycosylation, which emphasizes that glycosylation plays a crucial role in correct functioning of the NMJ. The reduction of endplate AChR explains why the patients respond well to treatment with cholinesterase inhibitors. It is possible, however, that other proteins apart from AChR subunits might also be abnormally glycosylated in *DPAGT1* and *GFPT1* patients.

The protein glycosylation pathway is a multistep process involving many different proteins. Since mutations in two of the genes have already been shown to lead to the development of CMS, it is likely that disruption of other genes in the pathway might lead to the development of similar phenotypes. Future genetic testing will help identify the genes involved and the exact clinical features associated with the disruption of these genes. Another interesting avenue for investigation is to understand why the symptoms of *DPAGT1*- and *GFPT1*-associated CMS are limited to NMJ function, and how different mutations in the same gene (*DPAGT1*) can lead to the development of two very different phenotypes found in CMS and CDG1J. In particular, it will be interesting to compare protein stability, catalytic activity, and the degree of impairment of AChR glycosylation caused by these mutations.

Acknowledgments

K.B. is a fellow of the Wellcome Trust–funded OXION: Ion Channels and Disease Initiative. We are grateful for funding from the Medical Research Council, UK, the Muscular Dystrophy Campaign, and the Myasthenia Gravis Association.

Conflicts of interest

The authors declare no conflicts of interest.

References

1. Chaouch, A., D. Beeson, D. Hantai & H. Lochmuller 2012. 186th ENMC international workshop: congenital myasthenic syndromes 24–26 June 2011, Naarden, The Netherlands. *Neuromuscul. Disord.* **22:** 566–576.
2. Engel, A.G. 2012. Current status of the congenital myasthenic syndromes. *Neuromuscul. Disord.* **22:** 99–111.
3. Senderek, J. *et al.* 2011. Hexosamine biosynthetic pathway mutations cause neuromuscular transmission defect. *Am. J. Hum. Genet.* **88:** 162–172.
4. Guergueltcheva, V. *et al.* 2012. Congenital myasthenic syndrome with tubular aggregates caused by GFPT1 mutations. *J. Neurol.* **259:** 838–850.
5. Belaya, K. *et al.* 2012. Mutations in DPAGT1 cause a limb-girdle congenital myasthenic syndrome with tubular aggregates. *Am. J. Hum. Genet.* **91:** 193–201.
6. Bretthauer, R.K. 2009. Structure, expression, and regulation of UDP-GlcNAc: dolichol phosphate GlcNAc-1-phosphate transferase (DPAGT1). *Curr. Drug Targets* **10:** 477–482.
7. Larkin, A. & B. Imperiali. 2011. The expanding horizons of asparagine-linked glycosylation. *Biochemistry* **50:** 4411–4426.
8. Lehle, L., S. Strahl & W. Tanner. 2006. Protein glycosylation, conserved from yeast to man: a model organism helps elucidate congenital human diseases. *Angew. Chem. Int. Ed. Engl.* **45:** 6802–6818.
9. Haeuptle, M.A. & T. Hennet. 2009. Congenital disorders of glycosylation: an update on defects affecting the biosynthesis of dolichol-linked oligosaccharides. *Hum. Mutat.* **30:** 1628–1641.
10. Schollen, E. *et al.* 2000. Genomic organization of the human phosphomannose isomerase (MPI) gene and mutation analysis in patients with congenital disorders of glycosylation type Ib (CDG-Ib). *Hum. Mutat.* **16:** 247–252.
11. Lefeber, D.J. *et al.* 2009. Deficiency of Dol-P-Man synthase subunit DPM3 bridges the congenital disorders of glycosylation with the dystroglycanopathies. *Am. J. Hum. Genet.* **85:** 76–86.
12. Zhu, X.Y. & M.A. Lehrman. 1990. Cloning, sequence, and expression of a cDNA encoding hamster UDP-GlcNAc: dolichol phosphate N-acetylglucosamine-1-phosphate transferase. *J. Biol. Chem.* **265:** 14250–14255.
13. Marek, K.W., I.K. Vijay & J.D. Marth. 1999. A recessive deletion in the GlcNAc-1-phosphotransferase gene results in peri-implantation embryonic lethality. *Glycobiology* **9:** 1263–1271.
14. Carrera, I.A., G. Matthijs, B. Perez & C.P. Cerda. 2012. DPAGT1-CDG: report of a patient with fetal hypokinesia phenotype. *Am. J. Med. Genet. A.* **158A:** 2027–2030.
15. Wu, X. *et al.* 2003. Deficiency of UDP-GlcNAc: Dolichol Phosphate N-Acetylglucosamine-1 Phosphate Transferase

(DPAGT1) causes a novel congenital disorder of glycosylation type Ij. *Hum. Mutat.* **22:** 144–150.

16. Wurde, A.E. *et al.* 2012. Congenital disorder of glycosylation type Ij (CDG-Ij, DPAGT1-CDG): extending the clinical and molecular spectrum of a rare disease. *Mol. Genet. Metab.* **105:** 634–41.

17. Martin, P.T. 2003. Glycobiology of the neuromuscular junction. *J. Neurocytol.* **32:** 915–929.

18. Ruff, R.L. 2011. Endplate contributions to the safety factor for neuromuscular transmission. *Muscle Nerve* **44:** 854–861.

19. Slater, C.R. 2008. Reliability of neuromuscular transmission and how it is maintained. *Handb. Clin. Neurol.* **91:** 27–101.

20. Croxen, R. *et al.* 2001. End-plate gamma- and epsilon-subunit mRNA levels in AChR deficiency syndrome due to epsilon-subunit null mutations. *Brain* **124:** 1362–1372.

21. Ohno, K. *et al.* 1997. Congenital myasthenic syndromes due to heteroallelic nonsense/missense mutations in the acetylcholine receptor epsilon subunit gene: identification and functional characterization of six new mutations. *Hum. Mol. Genet.* **6:** 753–766.

22. Slater, C.R. *et al.* 1997. Utrophin abundance is reduced at neuromuscular junctions of patients with both inherited and acquired acetylcholine receptor deficiencies. *Brain* **120**(Pt 9): 1513–1531.

23. Wanamaker, C.P., J.C. Christianson & W.N. Green. 2003. Regulation of nicotinic acetylcholine receptor assembly. *Ann. N.Y. Acad. Sci.* **998:** 66–80.

24. Gehle, V.M. & K. Sumikawa. 1991. Site-directed mutagenesis of the conserved N-glycosylation site on the nicotinic acetylcholine receptor subunits. *Brain Res. Mol. Brain Res.* **11:** 17–25.

25. Gehle, V.M., E.C. Walcott, T. Nishizaki & K. Sumikawa. 1997. N-glycosylation at the conserved sites ensures the expression of properly folded functional ACh receptors. *Brain Res. Mol. Brain Res.* **45:** 219–229.

26. Nomoto, H. *et al.* 1986. Carbohydrate structures of acetylcholine receptor from Torpedo californica and distribution of oligosaccharides among the subunits. *Eur. J. Biochem.* **157:** 233–242.

27. Pavlovicova, M., M. Novotova & I. Zahradnik. 2003. Structure and composition of tubular aggregates of skeletal muscle fibres. *Gen. Physiol. Biophys.* **22:** 425–440.

28. Schiaffino, S. 2012. Tubular aggregates in skeletal muscle: just a special type of protein aggregates? *Neuromuscul. Disord.* **22:** 199–207.

29. Beitz, E. 2000. T(E)Xtopo: shaded membrane protein topology plots in LAT(E)X2epsilon. *Bioinformatics* **16:** 1050–1051.

30. Larkin, M.A. *et al.* 2007. ClustalW and ClustalX version 2.0. *Bioinformatics* **23:** 2947–2948.

ANNALS OF THE NEW YORK ACADEMY OF SCIENCES

Issue: *Myasthenia Gravis and Related Disorders*

Synaptic basal lamina–associated congenital myasthenic syndromes

Ricardo A. Maselli,[1] Juan Arredondo,[1] Michael J. Ferns,[2] and Robert L. Wollmann[3]

[1]Department of Neurology. [2]Department of Anesthesiology, University of California, Davis, California. [3]Department of Pathology, University of Chicago, Chicago, Illinois

Address for correspondence: Ricardo A. Maselli, M.D., Department of Neurology, University of California Davis, 1515 Newton Court Room 510, Davis, CA 95618. ramaselli@ucdavis.edu

Proteins associated with the basal lamina (BL) participate in complex signal transduction processes that are essential for the development and maintenance of the neuromuscular junction (NMJ). Most important junctional BL proteins are collagens, such as collagen IV (α3–6), collagen XIII, and ColQ; laminins; nidogens; and heparan sulfate proteoglycans, such as perlecan and agrin. Mice lacking Colq ($Colq^{-/-}$), laminin β2 ($Lamb2^{-/-}$), or collagen XIII ($Col13a1^{-/-}$) show immature nerve terminals enwrapped by Schwann cell projections that invaginate into the synaptic cleft and decrease contact surface for neurotransmission. Human mutations in *COLQ*, *LAMB2*, and *AGRN* cause congenital myasthenic syndromes (CMSs) owing to deficiency of ColQ, laminin-β2, and agrin, respectively. In these syndromes the NMJ ultrastructure shows striking resemblance to that of mice lacking the corresponding protein; furthermore, the extracellular localization of mutant proteins may provide favorable conditions for replacement strategies based on gene therapy and stem cells.

Keywords: congenital myasthenic syndromes; basal lamina; ColQ; agrin; laminin β_2

The basal membrane (BM) of skeletal muscle, which was once thought to be a static structure that merely provides mechanical support to the muscle fiber, is currently viewed as a site of rich molecular interactions and key signal transduction processes involved in the development, regeneration, and maintenance of muscle.[1–4]

In strict terms, the name *basal lamina* (BL) refers only to the most internal layer of the BM,[2] but for the purpose of this short review, the terms *basal lamina* and *basal membrane* will be used interchangeably.

There are four major types of proteins at the synaptic BL of muscle: collagens, laminins, nidogens, and heparan sulfate proteoglycans (HSPG).

Collagens

The most abundant protein of the BL of muscle is the triple-helical collagen IV, which is formed by the variable assembly of six α chain isoforms (α1–α6). Collagen IV (α1)$_2$(α2) is the most abundant collagen protein of the extrasynaptic BL, whereas collagen IV (α3, α4, α5) and collagen IV (α5)$_2$(α6)

are primarily expressed at the NMJ.[5–7] Another collagen protein of the BL that plays a key role in the maturation of the NMJ is collagen XIII, which is a homotrimeric transmembrane protein with three collagenous regions and four interspaced noncollagenous domains.[8–10] An additional important collagen protein is the collagen-like "tail" ColQ, which is exclusively located at the synaptic BL where it assembles through its N-terminal proline-rich attachment domain (PRAD) to the C-terminal domain of the acetylcholinesterase (AChE) subunit to form the asymmetric AChE forms (Fig. 1).[11,12]

Laminins

The most abundant noncollagenous proteins of the BL are laminins, which are heterotrimers composed of α, β, and γ chains. At the NMJ the β2 and γ1 chains are invariably present in combination with α2, α4, or α5 chains that result in the formation of laminin-4 (α2β2γ1), −9 (α4β2γ1), and −11 (α5β2γ1), respectively.[13,14]

doi: 10.1111/j.1749-6632.2012.06807.x

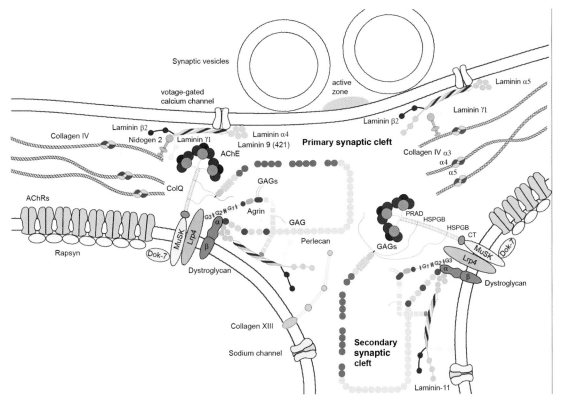

Figure 1. Diagram of the most important BL proteins at the NMJ (not drawn to scale). The LG2 domain of agrin, LG4 domain of laminin α-chains, and the C-terminus of perlecan bind to α-dystroglycan. Agrin binds through its LG3 domain to Lrp4 and through its C-terminus to the helical region of laminin. The GAGs attached to the N-terminus of perlecan bind to two HSPGB sites located at the collagen domain of ColQ, which is in turn attached through its N-terminal PRAD region to the AChE and through its C-terminal (CT) domain to MuSK. Finally, the laminin β2 chain binds through its C-terminus to presynaptic VGCC, and the laminin γ-chain binds to the C-terminus of nidogen-2, which connects through its N-terminus to collagen IV α-chains.

Nidogens

Collagens IV and laminin are both capable of self-assembly into two separate networks, which are linked to each other by another noncollagenous glycoprotein named *nidogen* (entactin), nidogen 2 being the isoform expressed at the NMJ.[15] The collagen IV and laminin networks are the backbone of the BM.

Heparan sulfate proteoglycans

Another group of important proteins of the BL are the HSPGs, such as perlecan, which are expressed throughout the muscle, and neural agrin (z+), which expressed exclusively at the NMJ outside of the central nervous system.[16] Collagen XVIII is another HSPG associated with the BL of skeletal muscle. Loss of collagen XVIII in *Caenorhabditis elegans* disrupts NMJ formation, but the role of

this protein at the mammal NMJ is currently uncertain.[17,18]

Other proteins associated with the BL

There are many other proteins associated with the BM, including fibronectin, tenascin, fibulins, and integrin receptors of laminins such as integrin $\alpha_7\beta_1$.[16] However, the precise role of these proteins at the vertebrate NMJ is unknown.

Protein interactions

Proteins associated with the muscle BL are rather large and several have longitudinal sizes that well exceed the transverse width of the primary synaptic cleft. Many BL proteins are capable of engaging in multiple interactions with other proteins of the extracellular matrix (ECM) as well as with cell-adhesion molecules and surface receptors that participate in complex intracellular signaling pathways. As an example, the C-terminal region of laminin β2 chain binds to presynaptic voltage-gated calcium channels (VGCC),[19,20] while the laminin α chain binds through its laminin globular (LG), such as domain 4 (LG4), to postsynaptic α-dystroglycan (DG) and through its LG1–3 domains to integrin cell surface receptors (Fig. 1).[21,22] The LG2 region of agrin and the C-terminus of perlecan also bind to α-DG and connect through the transmembrane β-DG with the intracellular cytoskeleton.[23] Agrin also binds through its N-terminus to the α-helical region of laminin and through its LG3 domain to its coreceptor Lrp4, which along with muscle-specific kinase (MuSK) and Dok-7 constitutes a fundamental signaling pathway for the development and maintenance of the NMJ.[24,25] In addition, two of the three N-terminal glycosaminoglycan (GAG) attachments of perlecan bind to two heparan-sulfate proteoglycan binding (HSPGB) sites located at the ColQ collagen domain, which is in turn attached through its C-terminal domain to MuSK.[26,27] There are many other important interactions between BL proteins among themselves and with cell surface receptors, including the binding of nidogen-2 to collagen IV, collagen XIII, perlecan, and the laminin γ chain and the binding of perlecan to laminins, fibronectin, collagen IV, collagen XIII, and AChE.[16,28] However, details about these protein interactions are beyond the scope of this short review.

Human diseases and mouse mutant phenotypes caused by deficiency of BL proteins of the NMJ

Many BL proteins present at the NMJ, such as laminin β2, collagen IV α3–6, perlecan, and nidogens, are also present at the BL of other tissues. As expected, human diseases caused by deficiencies of these proteins and the corresponding mouse mutant phenotypes often involve a broad spectrum of anomalies, including muscular, renal, cardiovascular, ocular, auditory, skeletal, and neurological abnormalities (Table 1). For instance, human mutations in *COL4A5* result in X-linked Alport syndrome, which is associated with glomerulonephritis (GNT), sensory-neural hearing loss, and often ocular abnormalities.[29–31] Although, myasthenic symptoms are not part of Alport syndrome, *COL4A5*[−/Y] mouse mutants, which lack α3–6 chains, show a large percentage of aberrant NMJs with pre- and postsynaptic abnormalities.[7] As another example, human mutations in *LAMB2* result in autosomal recessive (AR) Pierson syndrome, which involves renal and ocular anomalies.[32,33] However, *LAMB2* mutations can also result in congenital myasthenic syndrome (CMS) [34] and a wide range of additional clinical manifestations.[35]

In contrast, human mutations in *HSPG2*, the gene that encodes perlecan, do not cause CMSs or renal abnormalities but result in Schwartz–Jampel syndrome (SJS), which is a syndrome characterized by skeletal chondrodysplasia and continuous muscle discharges or neuromyotonia, presumably due to preterminal nerve dysmyelination leading to axonal depolarization and increased nerve excitability.[36–38]

A distinctive combination of pathological manifestations is linked to abnormalities in *LAMA4*, the gene that encodes laminin α4. In humans, mutations in *LAMA4* have been reported to cause cardiomyopathy;[39] whereas in mice, deficiency of laminin α4 results not only in cardiomyopathy and progressive glomerular sclerosis,[40,41] but also in a peculiar loss of precise apposition of presynaptic active zones to secondary synaptic clefts at the NMJ.[42,43] Deficiency of laminin α2 in humans and mice result in merosin-deficient congenital muscular dystrophy,[44–46] and pre- and postsynaptic defects of the NMJ have been reported in α2–deficient mice (i.e., missing laminin-4).[47]

On the other hand, knockout models of α5 and γ1 are lethal, and there are no known disease-causing mutations in genes encoding these laminin chains in humans.[48,49] Similarly, no mutations leading to human disease have ever been reported in genes encoding nidogen 2 or collagen XIII despite the fact that mice deficient in these proteins showed functional and structural abnormalities of the NMJ.[15,50]

As expected, deficiency of BL proteins expressing exclusively at the NMJ, like ColQ and agrin, result in disorders characterized only by functional and structural abnormalities of the NMJ.

Congenital myasthenic syndromes

To date mutations in genes encoding only three proteins of the synaptic BL have been identified as the cause of human CMSs (Table 2).[34,54,55] These three proteins, ColQ, laminin β2, and agrin, are associated with moderate-to-severe phenotypes in the

Table 1. Most important BL proteins of the NMJ and the human diseases and mouse mutant phenotypes related to these proteins

Gene	Protein	Human disease	Main clinical manifestations	Severity and phenotype of deficient mouse	NMJ defect	Role at the NMJ
COLQ	ColQ	Deficiency of endplate AChE	Muscle weakness	Moderate, neuro-muscular	Yes	Clustering of AChE and synaptic differentiation
LAMB2	Laminin β2	Pierson syndrome	Nephrosis, ocular deficit and muscle weakness	Severe, renal and neuro-muscular	Yes	Postnatal differentiation
AGRN	Agrin	Deficiency of agrin	Muscle weakness	Severe, neuro-muscular	Yes	Postsynaptic stabilization and maintenance
COL4A3	Collagen IV α3	Alport syndrome (AR)	GNT with hearing and ocular deficit	Severe, renal	Not reported	Synaptic maintenance
COL4A4	Collagen IV α4[a]	Alport syndrome (AR)	GNT with hearing and ocular deficit	Severe, renal	Not reported	Synaptic maintenance
COL4A5	Collagen IV α5	Alport syndrome (x-link)	GNT with hearing and ocular deficit	Severe, renal	Yes	Synaptic maintenance
COL4A6	Collagen IV α6	Alport syndrome (x-link)	GNT, hearing and ocular deficit plus diffuse leio-myomatosis[51]	Viable and fertile	Not reported	Synaptic maintenance
NID1	Nidogen 1	Not reported	–	Seizure-like behavior[52]	Not reported	Not reported
NID2	Nidogen 2	Not reported	–	Viable and fertile[15]	Yes	Maturation and maintenance
COL13A1	Collagen XIII	Not reported	–	Viable and fertile, but weak	Yes	Postsynaptic maturation
HSPG2	Perlecan	Schwartz–Jampel syndrome (SJS), dyssegmental dysplasia	Yes	Lethal, or SJS and chondro-dysplasia	Yes	Localization of AChE
LAMA2	Laminin α2	Merosin-deficiency muscular dystrophy	Muscle weakness	Severe, muscular dystrophy	Fold dysgenesis and nerve detach-ment	Synaptic and extra synaptic differentiation

Continued

Table 1. *Continued*

Gene	Protein	Human disease	Main clinical manifesta-tions	Severity and phenotype of deficient mouse	NMJ defect	Role at the NMJ
LAMA4	Laminin α4	Cardiomyopathy	Cardiac dysfunction	Progressive glomerular fibrosis, cardio-myopathy	Yes	Apposition of specialized presynaptic with postsynaptic structures
LAMA5	Laminin α5	Not reported	–	Lethal, polycystic kidney disease[53]	Not reported	Presynaptic differentiation and Schwann-cell repelling
LAMC1	Laminin γ1	Not reported	–	Lethal	Not reported	Not reported

[a]Absent in COL4A3[−/−] and COL4A5[−/Y] mutants.[7]

NOTE: Columns 1 and 2 list the most important genes and proteins associated with the BL of the NMJ. Columns 3 and 4 describe the human disease and the clinical manifestations. Columns 5 to 7 depict the phenotypes of corresponding animal models, the structure of the NMJ in these models, and the most important function of the affected proteins.

corresponding mouse-deficient mutants. Homozygous agrin-deficient mice develop normally throughout fetal life, but die in utero or are stillborn.[56] In contrast, laminin β2–deficient mice appear normal during the first few days after birth, but after the first week of life develop progressive weakness and proteinuria and die within the first four weeks of life.[57] Finally, the phenotype of Colq-deficient mice is moderate, and providing these animals receive proper amounts of food and water, the majority reach adulthood. However, they are unfertile and underweight and show weakness and jerking movements.[58]

Common pathogenic mechanisms

Human synaptic CMSs and corresponding mouse-deficient mutants share a number of structural and functional abnormalities of the NMJ that, although not totally specific, distinguish them from other types of CMSs and from other disorders of neuromuscular transmission (Table 2). The classical ultrastructural abnormalities of synaptic CMSs include reduction of the axon terminal size, partial encasement of the nerve endings by Schwann cells, focal simplification of postsynaptic folds with widening of the primary synaptic cleft, and invasion of

the synaptic cleft by the processes of Schwann cells (Fig. 2). Importantly, the simplification of the postsynaptic folds in synaptic CMSs is usually focal as opposed to generalized, as it is in postsynaptic CMS due to deficiency of AChR epsilon subunit or rapsyn. The changes described above are most prominent in deficiency of laminin β2 but are also present in varied degree in deficiency of endplate AChE and agrin.[34,54,55,59] However, they can also be occasionally encountered in other CMSs.[60] In addition, in deficiency of endplate AChE, there are subsynaptic degenerative abnormalities, including autophagic vacuoles, dilated sarcotubular elements, increased lipid droplets, and degenerating nuclei, which are often referred to as *endplate myopathy*.[54,61]

Findings of endplate myopathy are classically seen in experimental models of acute inhibition of the AChE.[62,63] However, these pathologic changes do not result from the inactivation of the AChE per se, but from the activation of lytic enzymes by the ion overload from the persistence of acetylcholine (ACh) at the synaptic cleft caused by the deficiency of AChE. Compelling evidence supporting this interpretation is the fact that subsynaptic degenerative changes are also seen, and are even more prominent than in deficiency of AChE, in the slow-channel

Table 2. Clinical features and pathophysiologic findings of synaptic BL–associated CMS

Human CMS	Deficiency of laminin β2	Deficiency of endplate acetylcholinesterase	Deficiency of agrin
Gene	*LAMB2*	*COLQ*	*AGRN*
Extraneurological manifestations	Yes, renal and ocular anomalies (Pierson syndrome)	No	No
Involvement of external ocular muscles	Variable	Variable	Mild
Respiratory insufficiency	Yes	Yes	Yes
Nerve terminal size	Reduced	Reduced	Reduced
Synaptic vesicle density	Decreased	Normal or increased	Normal or increased
Encasement by Schwann cell	Severe	Moderate	Mild to moderate
Invasion of synaptic cleft by Schwann cell processes	Severe	Moderate	Mild or absent
Width of primary and secondary synaptic cleft	Increased	Increased	Increased
Focal postsynaptic fold simplification	Moderate	Moderate	Mild
Degenerative changes	not reported	Yes, subsynaptic vacuoles consistent with endplate myopathy	Yes, myelin figures in nerve terminals and subsynaptic vacuoles
MEPP frequencies	Decreased	Decreased	Decreased
EPP quantal content	Decreased	Decreased	Decreased
MEPPs	Low amplitude	Low or normal amplitude with increased duration	Low or normal amplitude
Response to pyridostigmine	Poor	Poor	Fair

CMS where the AChE expression is normal and the ion-overload results from prolonged openings of the AChR ion channel.[64,65] It was originally thought that the reduction of size and the nerve terminal encasement by the Schwann cell in AChE deficiency was a secondary mechanism to protect the endplate from ion overload.[54] However, the presynaptic changes observed in AChE deficiency are also present in other synaptic CMSs that have no impaired AChE function.[34,59] Thus, the presynaptic changes of synaptic CMSs may represent a common reactive process to a broad range of pathologic insults. Finally, even if the release of AChE is ameliorated by the reduction in size and encasement of nerve terminals, evidence of endplate myopathy is often striking in some human cases of deficiency of endplate AChE (Fig. 3).

Failure of neuromuscular transmission

Compared with the failure of neuromuscular transmission observed in the majority of CMSs, which is either exclusively postsynaptic (e.g., deficiency of AChR epsilon subunit or rapsyn[66,67]) or predominantly postsynaptic (e.g., deficiency of MuSK or Dok-7[68,69]), the failure at the NMJ in synaptic CMSs is predominantly presynaptic. Nevertheless, in contrast to Lambert–Eaton myasthenic syndrome (LEMS) in which the presynaptic failure results from a decreased probability of synaptic vesicle release due to impaired entry of calcium into the nerve terminal, the presynaptic failure in synaptic CMSs is caused by a decreased number of synaptic vesicles immediately available for release and a decreased area of apposition between pre- and postsynaptic membranes.[34,54] A practical point

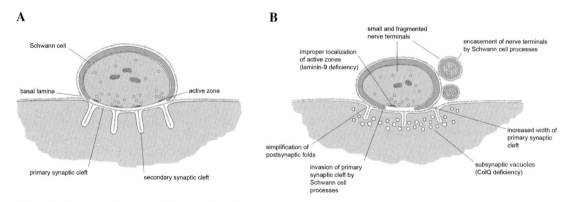

Figure 2. Common ultrastructural abnormalities of BL-associated CMS and their corresponding animal models.

derived from this observation is that in LEMS, high-frequency nerve stimulation causes accumulation of calcium at the nerve terminal leading to improvement of neuromuscular transmission, whereas in synaptic CMS, high-frequency nerve stimulation results in rapid depletion of synaptic vesicles and worsening of neuromuscular transmission. Thus, at fast stimulation rates, nerve terminals of synaptic CMSs and LEMS behave essentially in opposite ways.

Depletion of synaptic vesicles with fast stimulation rates would predictably be most severe in human disease and animal models caused by laminin β2 deficiency because, due to the concomitant deficiency of laminin-9 and laminin-11—and consequently laminins α4 and α5—the density of synaptic vesicles at the nerve terminal is diminished and active zones are not properly aligned with secondary synaptic clefts.[5,47] In contrast, in AChE and agrin deficiency, the density of synaptic vesicles is either normal or increased,[54,59] albeit insufficiently to compensate the underlying presynaptic deficit.

Postsynaptic failure is present in all synaptic CMSs; however, with regard to AChE deficiency, there are at least four additional postsynaptic mechanisms that contribute to the frequency-dependent failure of neuromuscular transmission (Fig. 3). First, due to the fact that endplate potential (EPP) half-decay times are long and outlast the refractory period of the muscle fiber action potential, a single nerve stimulation, or the first stimulation of a train of stimuli, results in repetitive firing of action potentials, rendering the muscle fiber transiently unresponsive to the normal activation by the nerve.[70] Repetitive firing of action potentials often results in a peculiar abrupt decrement of compound muscle

action potential (CMAP) amplitudes during a train of stimuli, which is maximal at the second CMAP of the train and progressively recovers thereafter.[71] This is occasionally observed in Colq-deficient mice and may be, in part, responsible for the jerking movements of these animals. Second, because of the long EPP half-decay times, EPPs summate upon each other in a staircase fashion causing depolarization of the muscle membrane.[70–72] As a result of the progressive depolarization of the muscle membrane there is concomitant reduction of the driving force that results in a progressive reduction of EPP amplitudes. Third, depolarization of the muscle membrane not only leads to reduction of EPP amplitudes, but also it produces inactivation of sodium channels that interferes with the generation of action potentials in the muscle fibers. Fourth, because of the accumulation of ACh at the synaptic cleft during rapid activation, AChRs become desensitized lowering the probability of AChR ion channel opening and further reducing EPP amplitudes.

In human agrin deficiency, there is normal expression of endplate AChE and the density of synaptic vesicles is either normal or increased.[55,59] Thus, the mechanisms described above would not be expected to play a significant role, and that may explain a less impressive frequency-dependent depression of synaptic transmission in this syndrome.

CMS due to deficiency of endplate acetylcholinesterase

This is one of the first congenital myasthenic syndrome types that were fully described, and one of the first CMSs in which the underlying molecular genetic defect was elucidated.[54,73] Yet, owing to the multiple mechanisms that participate in the

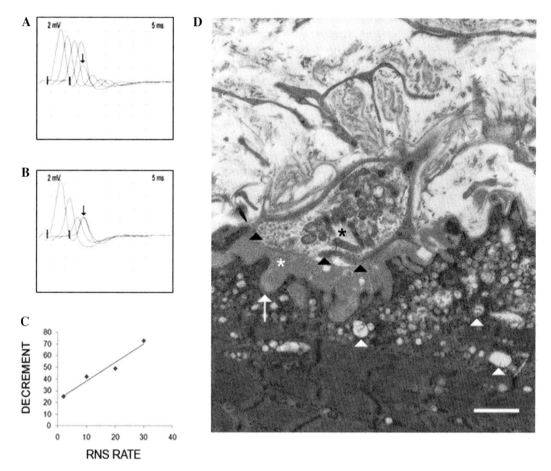

Figure 3. Electrodiagnostic findings and ultrastructural abnormalities of the NMJ in deficiency of endplate AChE. (A) Repetitive stimulation of the ulnar nerve at 2 Hz in a 16-year-old boy with AChE deficiency revealed 25% decrement of CMAP amplitudes. Arrows in A and B point at the second component of double CMAPs elicited by the first stimulus of the train. (B) Repetitive stimulation at 30 Hz showed a 72% decrement of CMAP amplitudes. (C) Decrement of CMAP amplitudes as a function of the frequency of stimulation in the same patient showing a linear increase of decrement with increasing rates of repetitive nerve stimulation. (D) Electron microscopy of a NMJ from a 9-year-old boy with AChE deficiency showing a nerve terminal (black asterisk) of reduced size, retracted from the postsynaptic membrane, and partially encased by the Schwann cell (black arrowheads). The primary synaptic cleft is widened and filled with debris material (white asterisk). There is also focal degeneration of postsynaptic folds (white arrows) and a large number of subsynaptic vacuoles (white arrowheads). The calibration mark represents 1 μm.

pathogenesis of this disorder, it remains one of the CMS most difficult to understand and most challenging to treat. Deficiency of AChE is a relatively frequent form of autosomal recessive CMS representing in our database 14% of a total of 70 cases of CMS all confirmed with genetic diagnosis and the majority studied with muscle biopsy. This percentage is similar to that reported by the Mayo Clinic based on a larger database, but slightly higher than the percentages reported by other centers.[74]

Deficiency of endplate AChE is caused by mutations in *COLQ*, a gene that generates multiple tran-

scripts variants encoding different isoforms of the triple helix ColQ protein.[73] The N-terminal domain of ColQ contains the PRAD region that assembles ColQ to the C-terminal region of the T splice variant of the AChE (AChE$_T$).[75]

In addition, ColQ has a collagenous domain that contains two heparin binding sites and a cysteine-rich C-terminal domain that interacts with MuSK and directly with the BL (Fig. 1).[27]

The globular (G) forms of the enzyme result from the self-assembly of AChE$_T$ in monomers (G1), dimers (G2), and tetramers (G4), while the variable assembly of $AChE_T$ tetramers to single, double, or triple ColQ alpha helices results in the asymmetric (A) forms A4, A8, and A12, respectively. [75,76] The different globular and asymmetric forms of AChE can be separated using sucrose density gradient centrifugation, followed by the Ellman assay in proteins extracted from muscle biopsy or from the lysate of cells cotransfected with $AChE_T$ and ColQ (wild type or mutant). [77,78]

Most human mutations in the N-terminal or collagenous domains of ColQ are nonsense or frameshift mutations that preclude the attachment of ColQ to $AChE_T$ or prevent triple helical assembly and result in the absence of asymmetric AChE forms in the sucrose density gradient. Conversely, at the C-terminal region, most defects are missense mutations that do not prevent the assembly of ColQ with $AChE_T$ or alter the sucrose density gradient. Most of these mutations impair the binding of ColQ to MuSK and the anchoring of the AChE to the BM, but the significance of the impaired binding of ColQ to MuSK is uncertain. [79–83]

Clinically, deficiency of endplate AChE is a disabling disorder that usually first manifests at birth or during infancy. Yet the onset of this disease can occur much later in life, particularly when the symptoms are mild. [60] Proximal muscle weakness associated with variable degree of ptosis, facial weakness, external ocular muscle involvement, and respiratory distress are the cardinal clinical features of this disease. The respiratory crises are usually associated with intercurrent infections as opposed to those in CMS that occurs because of choline acetyltransferase (*CHAT*) mutations. [84] In a review by Mihaylova *et al.*, some of the classical clinical features of AChE deficiency are described. For example, repetitive CMAP in response to a single stimulus may not be present, thus confusing the diagnosis and delaying appropriate treatment. [85]

Treatment of deficiency of endplate AChE is disappointing. Patients do not respond or worsen with AChE inhibitors and only moderately respond to sympathomimetic drugs such as ephedrine and albuterol. [86,87] Some patients improve with 3,4 diaminopyridine (DAP), but some patients are unable to tolerate the full dose of DAP. [88] Since depletion of synaptic vesicles, depolarization block, and endplate myopathy could theoretically all worsen with DAP, this drug should be administered with caution.

It has recently been reported that a single administration of adeno-associated virus serotype 8 (AAV8)-COLQ to the tail vein of Colq-deficient mice result in recovery of motor function and synaptic transmission. [89] This study suggests that replacement therapy with recombinant proteins may be a potentially effective modality of treatment for deficiency of endplate AChE and other types of synaptic CMS.

CMS due to deficiency of agrin

Agrin deficiency is a rare autosomal recessive syndrome with only two pedigrees reported to date in the literature and a recent abstract report of a new case. [55,59,90] The first pedigree reported consisted of two siblings from a consanguineous family with ptosis and intact external ocular movements, but with mild weakness of facial and hip-girdle muscles. [55] A second family involved a patient with more severe muscle weakness, mild external ocular involvement, and respiratory failure, and a younger sibling who presumably died from the same disease. [59] Microelectrode recordings performed in the patient from the second family were consistent with presynaptic failure of neuromuscular transmission. The ultrastructure of the NMJ common to both patients primarily involved the nerve terminal, which was either absent or reduced in size and partially encased by the Schwann cell. The density of synaptic vesicles was either normal [55] or increased. [59] In both cases, there was a bizarre enlargement of primary and secondary synaptic clefts and some degenerative changes in the nerve terminals and the subsynaptic regions.

Interestingly, all patients reported to date had mutations in the LG2 domain of agrin. The first pedigree carried the homozygous missense mutation G1709R, and the patient from the second pedigree was compound heterozygous for a null allele (Q353X) and the V1727F mutation. Expression studies showed that G1709R did not alter phosphorylation of MuSK or clustering of receptors, but when injected into rat muscles, it reproduced the changes of the NMJ observed in the patient. On the other hand, V1727F resulted in profound impairment of phosphorylation of MuSK and clustering of receptors in C2C12 myotubes and a curious increased in the affinity of agrin to alpha-DG mimicking nonneural (z-) agrin. The G1767D mutation reported in the abstract also resulted in reduced clustering of receptors. [90]

Patients identified with agrin mutations responded poorly to pharmacologic interventions, with the exception of some improvement with ephedrine in the patient from the first pedigree and with pyridostigmine bromide in the patient from the second pedigree.

CMS due to deficiency of laminin β2

Laminin β2 deficiency is a rare and severe form of autosomal recessive CMS with only two well-documented cases to date.[34,60] The disease has been observed in rare long-term survivors of congenital nephrosis as part of Pierson disease, which is itself a rare disorder.[32,33] The disease was originally described in a patient with biallelic truncation mutations in *LAMB2*, who had a long survival due to a highly compatible renal transplant from her father.[34] While the genetic defect in this patient provided a clear explanation for the neuromuscular disorder, why some, but not all long-term survivors with Pierson syndrome develop this disease is actually unknown.

The disease is clinically characterized by proximal and facial weakness with variable involvement of external ocular movements and respiratory failure. Electrodiagnostic studies have shown a decrement of CMAP amplitudes to repetitive nerve stimulation, with marked worsening at fast rates of stimulation.

Endplate studies showed severe reduction of MEPP frequencies and EPP quantal content, with moderate reduction of MEPP amplitudes and normal MEPP half-decay times. The nerve terminals showed decreased size and density of synaptic vesicles, and partial or complete encasement by the Schwann cell. The postsynaptic membranes were simplified and the synaptic cleft was partially invaded by processes of the Schwann cell. The physiologic and structural changes were strikingly similar to those described in laminin β2–deficient mice.[57,91,92] Treatment of this syndrome with AChE inhibitors is ineffective, and similar to deficiency of AChE, may be potentially dangerous. However, the originally reported case showed sustained benefit from treatment with DAP.[34] The mechanism by which DAP improved symptoms in this case is unclear, but it may be related to the well-known fact that DAP increases the nerve terminal release of ACh, which was severely reduced in this patient.

Conflicts of interest

The authors declare no conflicts of interest.

References

1. Colognato, H. & P.D. Yurchenco. 2000. Form and function: the laminin family of heterotrimers. *Dev. Dyn. Jun.* **218**: 213–234.
2. Sanes, J.R. 2003. The basement membrane/basal lamina of skeletal muscle. *J. Biol. Chem.* **278**: 12601–12604.
3. Campbell, K.P. & J.T. Stull. 2003. Skeletal muscle basement membrane-sarcolemma-cytoskeleton interaction minireview series. *Biol. Chem.* **278**: 12599–12600.
4. Yurchenco P.D. & B.L. Patton. 2009. Developmental and pathogenic mechanisms of basement membrane assembly. *Curr. Pharm. Des.* **15**: 1277–1294.
5. Sanes, J.R. *et al.* 1990. Molecular heterogeneity of basal laminae: isoforms of laminin and collagen IV at the neuromuscular junction and elsewhere. *J. Cell Biol.* **111**: 1685–1699.
6. Miner, J.H. & J.R. Sanes. 1994. Collagen IV alpha 3, alpha 4, and alpha 5 chains in rodent basal laminae: sequence, distribution, association with laminins, and developmental switches. *J. Cell Biol.* **127**: 879–891.
7. Fox, M.A. *et al.* 2007. Distinct target-derived signals organize formation, maturation, and maintenance of motor nerve terminals. *Cell* **129**: 179–193.
8. Hägg, P. *et al.* 1998. Type XIII collagen is identified as a plasma membrane protein. *J. Biol. Chem.* **273**: 15590–15597.
9. Peltonen, S. *et al.* 1999. A novel component of epidermal cell-matrix and cell-cell contacts: transmembrane protein type XIII collagen. *J. Invest. Dermatol.* **113**: 635–642.
10. Snellman, A. *et al.* 2000. Type XIII collagen forms homotrimers with three triple helical collagenous domains and its association into disulfide-bonded trimers is enhanced by prolyl 4-hydroxylase. *J. Biol. Chem.* **275**: 8936–8944.
11. Massoulié, J. *et al.* 1998. Acetylcholinesterase: C-terminal domains, molecular forms and functional localization. *J. Physiol. Paris* **92**: 183–190.
12. Rotundo, R.L. 2008. Assembly and regulation of acetylcholinesterase at the vertebrate neuromuscular junction. *Chem. Biol. Interact.* **175**: 26–29.
13. Patton, B.L. *et al.* 1997. Distribution and function of laminins in the neuromuscular system of developing, adult, and mutant mice. *J. Cell Biol.* **139**: 1507–1521.
14. Miner, J.H. *et al.* 2006. Transgenic isolation of skeletal muscle and kidney defects in laminin beta2 mutant mice: implications for Pierson syndrome. *Development* **133**: 967–975.
15. Fox, M.A. *et al.* 2008. A synaptic nidogen: developmental regulation and role of nidogen-2 at the neuromuscular junction. *Neural. Dev.* **25**: 3–24.
16. Singhal, N. & P.T. Marin. 2011. Role of extracellular matrix proteins and their receptors in the development of the vertebrate neuromuscular junction. *Dev. Neurobiol.* **71**: 982–1005.

17. Ackley, B.D. *et al.* 2003. The basement membrane components nidogen and type XVIII collagen regulate organization of neuromuscular junctions in Caenorhabditis elegans. *J. Neurosci.* **23:** 3577–3587.

18. Werle, M.J. 2009. *Developmental Neurobiology*. Academic Press. London.

19. Nishimune, H., J.R. Sanes & S.S. Carlson. 2004. A synaptic laminin-calcium channel interaction organizes active zones in motor nerve terminals. *Nature* **432:** 580–587.

20. Nishimune, H. 2012. Molecular mechanism of active zone organization at vertebrate neuromuscular junctions. *Mol. Neurobiol.* **45:** 1–16.

21. Munoz, J., Y. Zhou & H.W. Jarrett. 2010. LG4–5 domains of laminin-211 binds alpha-dystroglycan to allow myotube attachment and prevent anoikis. *J. Cell Physiol.* **222:** 111–119.

22. Suzuki, N. *et al.* 2010. Identification of alpha-dystroglycan binding sequences in the laminin alpha2 chain LG4–5 module. *Matrix Biol.* **29:** 143–151.

23. Hohenester, E. *et al.* 1999. The crystal structure of a laminin G-like module reveals the molecular basis of alpha-dystroglycan binding to laminins, perlecan, and agrin. *Mol. Cell.* **4:** 783–792.

24. Kim, N. *et al.* 2008. Lrp4 is a receptor for Agrin and forms a complex with MuSK. *Cell* **135:** 334–342.

25. Zhang, B. *et al.* 2008. LRP4 serves as a coreceptor of agrin. *Neuron* **60:** 285–297.

26. Rotundo, R.L. *et al.* 2008. Assembly and regulation of acetylcholinesterase at the vertebrate neuromuscular junction. *Chem. Biol. Interact.* **175:** 26–29.

27. Cartaud, A. *et al.,* 2004. MuSK is required for anchoring acetylcholinesterase at the neuromuscular junction. *J. Cell. Biol.* **165:** 505–515.

28. LeBleu, V.S., B. Macdonald & R. Kalluri. 2007. Structure and function of basement membranes. *Exp. Biol. Med.* **232:** 1121–1129.

29. Kashtan, C.E. 2009. Familial hematuria. *Pediatr. Nephrol.* **24:** 1951–1958.

30. Miner, J.H. 2011. Organogenesis of the kidney glomerulus: focus on the glomerular basement membrane. *Organogenesis* **7:** 75–82.

31. Rheault, M.N. *et al.* 2012. Women and Alport syndrome. *Pediatr. Nephrol.* **27:** 41–46.

32. Zenker, M. *et al.* 2004. Human laminin beta2 deficiency causes congenital nephrosis with mesangial sclerosis and distinct eye abnormalities. *Hum. Mol. Genet.* **13:** 2625–2632.

33. Zenker, M. *et al.* 2004. Congenital nephrosis, mesangial sclerosis, and distinct eye abnormalities with microcoria: an autosomal recessive syndrome. *Am. J. Med. Genet. A.* **130:** 138–145.

34. Maselli, R.A. *et al.* 2009. Mutations in LAMB2 causing a severe form of synaptic congenital myasthenic syndrome. *J. Med. Genet.* **46:** 203–208.

35. Matejas, V. *et al.* 2010. Mutations in the human laminin beta2 (LAMB2) gene and the associated phenotypic spectrum. *Hum. Mutat.* **31:** 992–1002.

36. Nicole, S. *et al.* 2000. Perlecan, the major proteoglycan of basement membranes, is altered in patients with Schwartz–Jampel syndrome (chondrodystrophic myotonia). *Nat. Genet.* **26:** 480–483.

37. Arikawa-Hirasawa, E. *et al.* 2002. Structural and functional mutations of the perlecan gene cause Schwartz–Jampel syndrome, with myotonic myopathy and chondrodysplasia. *Am. J. Hum. Genet.* **70:** 1368–1375.

38. Bangratz, M. *et al.* 2012. A mouse model of Schwartz–Jampel syndrome reveals myelinating Schwann cell dysfunction with persistent axonal depolarization in vitro and distal peripheral nerve hyperexcitability when perlecan is lacking. *Am. J. Pathol.* **180:** 2040–2055.

39. Knöll, R. *et al.* 2007. Laminin-alpha4 and integrin-linked kinase mutations cause human cardiomyopathy via simultaneous defects in cardiomyocytes and endothelial cells. *Circulation* **116:** 515–525.

40. Wang, J. *et al.* 2006. Cardiomyopathy associated with microcirculation dysfunction in laminin alpha4 chain-deficient mice. *J. Biol. Chem.* **281:** 213–220.

41. Abrass, C.K., K.M. Hansen & B.L. Patton. 2010. Laminin alpha4-null mutant mice develop chronic kidney disease with persistent overexpression of platelet-derived growth factor. *Am. J. Pathol.* **176:** 839–849.

42. Nishimune H et al. 2008. Laminins promote postsynaptic maturation by an autocrine mechanism at the neuromuscular junction. *J. Cell Biol.* **182:** 1201–1215.

43. Patton, B.L. *et al.* 2001. Properly formed but improperly localized synaptic specializations in the absence of laminin alpha4. *Nat. Neurosci.* **4:** 597–604.

44. Xu, H. *et al.* 1994. Murine muscular dystrophy caused by a mutation in the laminin alpha 2 (Lama2) gene. *Nat. Genet.* **8:** 297–302.

45. Helbling-Leclerc, A. *et al.* 1995. Mutations in the laminin alpha 2-chain gene (LAMA2) cause merosin-deficient congenital muscular dystrophy. *Nat. Genet.* **11:** 216–218.

46. Naom, I.S. *et al.* 1997. Refinement of the laminin alpha2 chain locus to human chromosome 6q2 in severe and mild merosin deficient congenital muscular dystrophy. *J. Med. Genet.* **34:** 99–104.

47. Patton, B.L. 2000. Laminins of the neuromuscular system. *Microsc. Res. Tech.* **51:** 247–261.

48. Miner, J.H., J. Cunningham & J.R. Sanes. 1998. Roles for laminin in embryogenesis: exencephaly, syndactyly, and placentopathy in mice lacking the laminin α5 chain. *J. Cell Biol.* **143:** 1713–1723.

49. Smyth, N. *et al.* 1999. Absence of basement membranes after targeting the LAMC1 gene results in embryonic lethality due to failure of endoderm differentiation. *J. Cell Biol.* **144:** 151–160.

50. Latvanlehto A. *et al.* 2010. Muscle-derived collagen XIII regulates maturation of the skeletal neuromuscular junction. *J. Neurosci.* **30:** 12230–12241.

51. Heidet, L. *et al.* 1995. Deletions of both alpha 5(IV) and alpha 6(IV) collagen genes in Alport syndrome and in Alport syndrome associated with smooth muscle tumours. *Hum. Mol. Genet.* **4:** 99–108.

52. Dong, L. *et al.* 2002. Neurologic defects and selective disruption of basement membranes in mice lacking entactin-1/nidogen-1. *Lab. Invest.* **82:** 1617–1630.

53. Shannon, M.B. *et al.* 2006. Hypomorphic mutation in the mouse laminin α5 gene (Lama5) causes polycystic kidney disease. *J. Am. Soc. Nephrol.* **17:** 1913–1922.

54. Engel, A.G., E.H. Lambert & M.R. Gomez. 1977. New myasthenic syndrome with end-plate acetylcholinesterase deficiency, small nerve terminals, and reduced acetylcholine release. *Ann. Neurol.* **1:** 315–330.

55. Huzé, C. *et al.* 2009. Identification of an agrin mutation that causes congenital myasthenia and affects synapse function. *Am. J. Hum. Genet.* **85:** 155–167.

56. Gautam, M. *et al.* 1996. Defective neuromuscular synaptogenesis in agrin-deficient mutant mice. *Cell* **85:** 525–535.

57. Noakes, P.G. *et al.* 1995. Aberrant differentiation of neuromuscular junctions in mice lacking s-laminin/laminin beta 2. *Nature* **374:** 258–262.

58. Feng, G. *et al.* 1999. Genetic analysis of collagen Q: roles in acetylcholinesterase and butyrylcholinesterase assembly and in synaptic structure and function. *J. Cell Biol.* **144:** 1349–1360.

59. Maselli, R.A. *et al.* 2012. LG2 agrin mutation causing severe congenital myasthenic syndrome mimics functional characteristics of non-neural (z-) agrin. *Hum. Genet.* **131:** 1123–1135.

60. Engel, A.G. 2012. Current status of the congenital myasthenic syndromes. *Neuromusc. Disord.* **22:** 99–111.

61. Feng, G. *et al.* 1999. Genetic analysis of collagen Q: roles in acetylcholinesterase and butyrylcholinesterase assembly and in synaptic structure and function. *J. Cell Biol.* **144:** 1349–1360.

62. Laskowski, M.B., W.H. Olson & W.D. Dettbarn. 1975. Ultrastructural changes at the motor end-plate produced by an irreversible cholinesterase inhibitor. *Exp. Neurol.* **47:** 290–306.

63. Salpeter, M.M. *et al.* 1979. End-plates after esterase inactivation in vivo: correlation between esterase concentration, functional response and fine structure. *J. Neurocytol.* **8:** 95–115.

64. Engel, A.G. *et al.* 1982. A newly recognized congenital myasthenic syndrome attributed to a prolonged open time of the acetylcholine-induced ion channel. *Ann. Neurol.* **11:** 553–569.

65. Vohra, B.P. *et al.* 2004. Focal caspase activation underlies the endplate myopathy in slow-channel syndrome. *Ann. Neurol.* **55:** 347–352.

66. Engel, A.G. *et al.* 1996. End-plate acetylcholine receptor deficiency due to nonsense mutations in the epsilon subunit. *Ann. Neurol.* **40:** 810–817.

67. Ohno, K. *et al.* 2002. Rapsyn mutations in humans cause endplate acetylcholine-receptor deficiency and myasthenic syndrome. *Am. J. Hum. Genet.* **70:** 875–885.

68. Anderson, J.A. *et al.* 2008. Variable phenotypes associated with mutations in DOK7. *Muscle Nerve* **37:** 448–456.

69. Maselli, R.A. *et al.* 2010. Mutations in MUSK causing congenital myasthenic syndrome impair MuSK-Dok-7 interaction. *Hum. Mol. Genet.* **19:** 2370–2379.

70. Maselli, R.A. & B.C. Soliven. 1991. Analysis of the organophosphate-induced electromyographic response to repetitive nerve stimulation: paradoxical response to edrophonium and D-tubocurarine. *Muscle Nerve* **14:** 1182–1188.

71. Maselli, R., J.H. Jacobsen & J.P. Spire. 1986. Edrophonium: an aid in the diagnosis of acute organophosphate poisoning. *Ann. Neurol.* **19:** 508–510.

72. Maselli, R.A. & C. Leung. 1993. Analysis of anticholinesterase-induced neuromuscular transmission failure. *Muscle Nerve* **16:** 548–553.

73. Ohno, K. *et al.* 1998. Human endplate acetylcholinesterase deficiency caused by mutations in the collagen-like tail subunit (ColQ) of the asymmetric enzyme. *Proc. Natl. Acad. Sci. USA* **95:** 9654–9659.

74. Chaouch, A. *et al.* 2012. 186th ENMC international workshop: congenital myasthenic syndromes 24–26 June 2011, Naarden, The Netherlands. *Neuromuscul. Disord.* **22:** 566–576.

75. Massoulié, J. 2002. The origin of the molecular diversity and functional anchoring of cholinesterases. *Neurosignals* **11:** 130–143.

76. Massoulié, J. & C.B. Millard. 2009. Cholinesterases and the basal lamina at vertebrate neuromuscular junctions. *Curr. Opin. Pharmacol.* **9:** 316–325.

77. Ellman, G.L. *et al.* 1961. Courtney KD, Andres V, FeatherStone RM. A new and rapid colorimetric determination of acetylcholinesterase activity. *Biochem. Pharmacol* **7:** 88–95.

78. Hall, Z.W. 1973. Multiple forms of acetylcholinesterase and their distribution in endplate and non-endplate regions of rat diaphragm muscle. *J. Neurobiol.* **4:** 343–361.

79. Ohno, K. *et al.* 2000. The spectrum of mutations causing end-plate acetylcholinesterase deficiency. *Ann. Neurol.* **47:** 162–170.

80. Donger, C. *et al.* 1998. Mutation in the human acetylcholinesterase-associated collagen gene, COLQ, is responsible for congenital myasthenic syndrome with endplate acetylcholinesterase deficiency (Type Ic). *Am. J. Hum. Genet.* **63:** 967–975.

81. Maselli, R. *et al.* 2003. Endplate (EP) acetylcholinesterase (AChE) deficiency due to COLQ mutations: missense mutations in the C-terminal do not prevent assembly of COLQ to the catalytic subunit. *Neurology* **60**(Suppl): A389.

82. Kimbell, L.M. *et al.* 2004. C-terminal and heparin-binding domains of collagenic tail subunit are both essential for anchoring acetylcholinesterase at the synapse. *J. Biol. Chem.* **279:** 10997–11005.

83. Arredondo *et al.* COOH-terminal COLQ mutants causing human deficiency of endplate acetylcholinesterase impair the interaction of ColQ with protein of the basal lamina. In preparation.

84. Ohno, K. *et al.* 2001. Choline acetyltransferase mutations cause myasthenic syndrome associated with episodic apnea in humans. *Proc. Natl. Acad. Sci. USA* **98:** 2017–2022.

85. Mihaylova, V. *et al.* 2008. Clinical and molecular genetic findings in COLQ-mutant congenital myasthenic syndromes. *Brain* **131:** 747–759.

86. Bestue-Cardiel, M. *et al.* 2005. Congenital endplate acetylcholinesterase deficiency responsive to ephedrine. *Neurology* **65:** 144–146.

87. Liewluck, T., D. Selcen & A.G. Engel. 2011. Beneficial effects of Albuterol in congenital endplate acetylcholinesterase deficiency and DOK-7 myasthenia. *Muscle Nerve* **44:** 789–794.

88. Guven, A., M. Demirci & B. Anlar. 2012. Recurrent COLQ mutation in congenital myasthenic syndrome. *Pediatr. Neurol.* **46:** 253–256.

89. Ito, M. *et al.* 2012. Protein-anchoring strategy for delivering acetylcholinesterase to the neuromuscular junction. *Mol. Ther.* **20:** 1384–1392.

90. Belaya, K., S. Finlayson, J. Cossins, W.W. Liu, S. Maxwell, J. Palace & D. Beeson. 2012. Identification of *DPAGT1* as a new gene in which mutations cause a congenital myasthenic syndrome. *Ann. N.Y. Acad. Sci.* **1275:** 29–35.

91. Knight, D. *et al.* 2003. Functional analysis of neurotransmission at β2-laminin deficient terminals. *J. Physiol.* **546:** 789–800.

92. Patton, B.L., A.Y. Chiu & J.R. Sanes. 1998. Synaptic laminin prevents glial entry into the synaptic cleft. *Nature* **393:** 698–701.

Ann. N.Y. Acad. Sci. ISSN 0077-8923

ANNALS OF THE NEW YORK ACADEMY OF SCIENCES

Issue: *Myasthenia Gravis and Related Disorders*

DOK7 congenital myasthenic syndrome

Jacqueline Palace

Clinical Neurology, John Radcliffe Hospital, Oxford University Hospitals NHS Trust, Oxford, United Kingdom

Address for correspondence: Dr. Jacqueline Palace, Department of Neurology, Level 3 West Wing, John Radcliffe Hospital, Headley Way, Oxford, OX3 9DU, UK. jacqueline.palace@ndcn.ox.ac.uk

Despite being a fairly recent discovery, DOK7 congenital myasthenic syndrome (CMS) is the third most common form of CMS in the United Kingdom. DOK7 is a postsynaptic protein associated with the AChR clustering pathway. In contrast to AChR deficiency due to epsilon subunit mutations, onset of DOK7 CMS tends to be later—ages two to three years—and in DOK7 CMS eye movements are usually spared and anticholinesterases can exacerbate the weakness. The typical phenotype of DOK7 CMS is of a limb girdle weakness with associated nonspecific myopathic features. The presence of stridor in early onset cases and the observation of tongue wasting may be specific clues. Worsening in adulthood is common, particularly affecting bulbar and respiratory function. Treatment with ephedrine or oral salbutamol can result in a slow, steady, and often dramatic improvement over months.

Background

The congenital myasthenic syndromes (CMSs) cover a heterogeneous group of genetic disorders affecting neuromuscular transmission. Currently, at least 15 genes and more than 300 different mutations have been associated with CMS, and the majority of these affect the postsynaptic neuromuscular junction structure and function.

The classical features of CMS include onset of weakness at birth or in infancy, worsening weakness with repetitive use or as the day goes on, commonly (but not always) a response to anticholinesterases, and relative stability throughout life (in contrast to some of its differential diagnoses). CMSs have an autosomal recessive mode of inheritance, with the exception of the slow channel syndrome which is dominantly inherited. Thus, a family history may aid diagnosis, and prevalence increases with parental consanguinity. CMS affects similar muscles to those affected in the acquired myasthenias including face, limb, bulbar, respiratory, and trunk muscles and, typically, causes ptosis and restricted eye movements. This review outlines the features of CMS caused by mutations in the *DOK7* gene and focuses on features that can differentiate it from other forms of CMS.

Genetics

DOK7 is a postsynaptic cytoplasmic protein that binds and activates muscle-specific tyrosine kinase, which in turn leads to Rapsyn-associated endplate AChR clustering and normal folding of the postsynaptic membrane.

In the United Kingdom, 92% of mutation-confirmed CMS cases are postsynaptic; DOK7 CMS was first described in 2006[1] and constitutes around 20% of the total. Around 65% of patients with DOK7 mutations have at least one copy of the common mutation[2] 1124_1127dupTGCC, which is located in the C-terminal domain and affects the ability of DOK7 to activate MuSK without preventing direct binding. However higher rates (80–90%) of this common mutation have been reported from other groups.[3–5]

Clinical phenotype

The features of DOK7 CMS from four studies have been summarized in Table 1; Table 2 lists the key features that can help differentiate it from other CMSs.

Onset and natural history

Patients with this form of CMS often present after infancy—around 18 months[2]—with walking

Table 1. Features of *DOK7* CMS[a]

Cohort:	Palace et al.[1, a]	Muller et al.[2]	Selcen et al.[3]	Ammar et al.[4]
Onset age (median and range)	18 months (0–5.5 years)	2 years (0–25 years)	1 year (fetal–5 years)	15 months (fetal–13 years)
Delayed walking age	0/15			0/15
Ptosis	94%	12/14	14/16	11/15
Asymmetry	64%			
EOM restricted	<20%	2/14	6/16 (mild in 5)	6/15
Facial weakness	83%	9/14	13/16	8/15
Bulbar symptoms	55%	7/14	11/16	9/15
Respiratory symptom	52%	10/14	13/16	11/15
Limb girdle pattern weakness	93% (and distal in 31%)	13/14	16/16 (and distal in 5)	15/15 (and distal in 12)
Clinical course:				
worsening	57%	10/14 (5 mild)	12/16	11/15
stable	22%	2/14 no progression		4/15 no progression
improving	21%	1/14		
Tongue wasting	53%	2		
Truncal weakness	37%			13/14
Neck weakness	66%			
Abnormal muscle biopsy	8/8		14/14	12/14
Response to:				
anticholinesterase	1↑[b], 6→, 5↓	7s-t↑only, l-t 6→, 4↓		1↑(+2s-t), 6→, 8↓
3,4-DAP	5↑, 4→, 3↓			6↑, 2→
ephedrine	5↑			1↑

s-t = short-term; l-t = long term.
[a]Updated information from 36 patients.
[b]Single DOK7 mutation subsequently identified as DPAGT1.

difficulties and, later, falls and difficulty running. Even those who have earlier symptoms often have a normal walking age milestone. Early symptoms include ptosis (which maybe recognized retrospectively), bulbar problems, and hypotonia. In a series of children with CMS, congenital stridor was only seen in those with DOK7 mutations, occurring in 6 of 11 DOK7 cases.[6] It was noteworthy that stri-

Table 2. Useful differentiating features of DOK7 CMS

Onset after infancy
Normal walking age
Limb-girdle phenotype without TA
Normal eye movements
Stridor
Tongue wasting
Associated nonspecific myopathy
Poor response to pyridostigmine ± 3,4-DAP

dor was associated with other bulbar symptoms but no other muscle weakness initially, and it often resolved; so this early history may not be apparent if diagnosed in adulthood. Stridor can occasionally occur in association with rapsyn and CHRNE fast-channel CMS, but it is uncommon and usually associated with other features of CMS. Onset of DOK7 CMS in the third decade has been reported in two siblings.[3]

Fluctuations are noted but often not the typical myasthenic worsening as the day goes on. Characteristically, patients describe worsening lasting weeks, although shorter exacerbations, such as premenstrual deteriorations, are described. The disease course has been described as variable, with some patients reporting improvement over time, some a stable course, and others reporting progression. The condition may worsen during puberty and then improve or remain stable in the second decade and

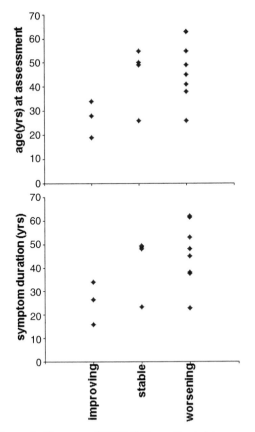

Figure 1. The course of DOK7 CMS according to (a) age examined and (b) disease duration from Palace *et al.*,[2] demonstrating a trend for progression to occur later in the disease process.

later, with progression lasting a few years or longer common. Thus, the course of disease may be related to the age of the patient and duration (Fig. 1), an observation supported by other cohorts.[3,5]

Pattern of weakness

The typical clinical picture of DOK7 CMS[2] includes a limb girdle pattern of weakness, although many patients also have distal weakness of the hands and ankle dorsiflexion. Ptosis is usual and often asymmetrical, and facial weakness can be severe associated with a "snarling smile." Truncal involvement is common. Bulbar and respiratory involvement is usual and often develops or progresses in adulthood. Because of pelvic girdle and truncal weakness, patients are classically described as having a waddling, sinuous gait, and spinal deformities such as scoliosis, kyphosis, and hyperlordosis are frequent.[3,5] Muscle atrophy is common but not specific, although tongue wasting (see Fig. 2) may be a help-

ful sign for directing genetic testing.[2] Contractures and hypermobility have been occasionally noted. Although this phenotype is the most commonly seen in DOK7 CMS it is not specific and overlaps with other forms of CMS, congenital myopathy, and early onset seronegative autoimmune MG. In contrast to CMS caused by mutations in the AChR subunits, eye movements are usually normal. Because rapysn CMS is also associated with a full range of eye movements, it is possible that the different innervation patterns in ocular muscle fibers make them less dependent on AChR clustering.

Neurophysiology

Most patients will show neurophysiological abnormalities, such as decrement on repetitive nerve stimulation or jitter, and block on single-fiber EMG. However, where weakness is limited to proximal muscle groups, repetitive muscle stimulation can be particularly sensitive.

Treatment

It was noticeable early on in the discovery of DOK7 CMS that these patients did not respond as expected to anticholinesterases and 3,4-DAP.[2] A minority noted a short-term improvement only with pyridostigmine, but the majority found it either had no effect or made them worse; 3,4-DAP appeared to help about half the patients. Of note, a few patients whose CMS was subsequently genetically confirmed as DOK7 related had been taking ephedrine because they found it beneficial. This has subsequently led to the documentation that either ephedrine[7] or oral salbutamol[8] can lead to a marked improvement in muscle strength and an even more dramatic effect on day-to-day function. However, this effect is delayed and improvement continues over months. Because ephedrine and oral salbutamol are rarely used and are not licensed for CMS, we recommend a cautious approach, which includes blood pressure monitoring and obtaining an ECG at the start and then intermittently thereafter. Some patients benefit from the addition of 3,4-DAP, although, again, the safety data on combining these therapies are limited. Salbutamol may be preferred to ephedrine because it is readily available, it is more familiar to physicians, and it may start to work a little more quickly; however, its use is sometimes limited by troublesome muscle cramps. Ephedrine appears well tolerated, although both drugs appear equally efficacious. An

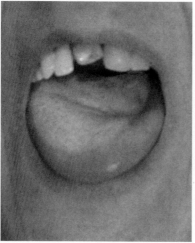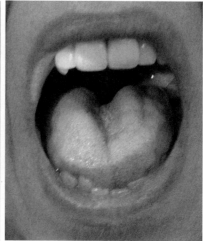

Figure 2. Two examples of tongue wasting in patients with DOK7 CMS.

immediate stimulant effect may be noted (and appreciated) by patients. Table 3 outlines the treatment regime.

Although the mechanism for the observed poor efficacy of anticholinesterases (and 3,4-DAP in some) is not clear, it may be related to the proposed inhibitory effect DOK7 has on AChR dispersion with increased cholinergic stimulation.

Evidence of an associated end-plate myopathy

In addition to the neurophysiological tests being consistent with a neuromuscular transmission de-

Table 3. Treatment regime

Ephedrine
  Start at dose 15 mg bd (adult)
  ECG and blood pressure monitoring baseline,
    +1–2 hr, one week, as required
  Review at six months and increase dose if no effect
    or positive effect stabilized
  Improvement can continue beyond six months
  May need dose increasing up to 30 mg tds
Salbutamol
  Start at dose of 4 mg bd
  Monitor as for ephedrine
  Improvement can continue beyond six months
May need dose increasing up to 8 mg bd
3,4-DAP but not pyridostigmine may be added
  cautiously where above not sufficient

---

fect, these patients usually have nonspecific myopathic features. Although creatine kinase is normal or only mildly elevated, standard electromyography shows myogenic changes in most patients tested, and the muscle biopsy may demonstrate predominance of type I and atrophy of type II fibers and lipidosis.[5] Electron microscopy does not demonstrate tubular aggregates, and analysis of neuromuscular junction structure has demonstrated small pre- and postsynaptic structures with normal density of AChR.[4,9] The development of a secondary endplate myopathy in DOK7 CMS might explain the progressive disease course and slow response to ephedrine and salbutamol, which probably act as endplate stabilizers. If this hypothesis is correct, treating early might reduce or prevent future deterioration.

Differential diagnoses

DOK7 CMS needs to be differentiated from other CMSs, and this is usually straightforward because of the availability of genetic testing. However, identifying intronic mutations, large deletions, and establishing pathogenicity of new mutations can be challenging and time consuming.

Late onset cases can be difficult to differentiate from the seronegative myasthenias, and patients may have been given a trial of immunomodulatory treatments and occasionally have even been thymectomized. Because of the associated myopathic features, differential diagnoses include congenital myopathy, muscular dystrophy, and metabolic and mitochondrial myopathies. In infants presenting with stridor and in young children with walking/running problems, the differential is broader still.

Conflicts of interest

The author declares no conflicts of interest.

References

1. Beeson, D., O. Higuchi, J. Palace, *et al*. 2006. Dok-7 mutations underlie a neuromuscular junction synaptopathy. *Science* **313:** 1975–1978.
2. Palace, J., D. Lashley, J. Newsom-Davis, *et al*. 2007. Clinical features of the DOK7 neuromuscular junction synaptopathy. *Brain* **130:** 1507–1515.
3. Muller, J.S., A. Herczegfalvi, J.J. Vilchez, *et al*. 2007. Phenotypical spectrum of DOK7 mutations in congenital myasthenic syndromes. *Brain* **130:** 1497–1506.
4. Selcen, D., M. Milone, X.M. Shen, *et al*. 2008. MD Dok-7 myasthenia: phenotypic and molecular genetic studies in 16 patients. *Ann. Neurol.* **64:** 71–87.
5. Ammar, A.B., F. Petit, N. Alexandri, *et al*. 2010. Phenotype genotype analysis in 15 patients presenting a congenital myasthenic syndrome due to mutations in DOK7. *J. Neurol.* **257:** 754–766.
6. Jephson, C.G., N.A. Mills, M.C. Pitt, *et al*. 2010. Congenital stridor with feeding difficulty as a presenting symptom of Dok7 congenital myasthenic syndrome. *Int. J. Ped. Otorhinolaryngol.* **74:** 991–994.
7. Lashley, D., J. Palace, S. Jayawant, *et al*. 2010. Ephedrine treatment in congenital myasthenic syndrome due to mutations in DOK7. *Neurology* **74:** 1517–1523.
8. Burke, G., A. Hiscock, A. Klein, *et al*. 2011. Salbutamol treatment in children with DOK7 congenital myasthenic syndrome. *Eur. J. Paed. Neurol.* **15**(Suppl 1)**:** 2 abstract.
9. Slater, C.R., P.R. Fawcett, T.J. Walls, *et al*. 2006. Pre- and post-synaptic abnormalities associated with impaired neuromuscular transmission in a group of patients with 'limb-girdle myasthenia'. *Brain* **129:** 2061–2076.

Ann. N.Y. Acad. Sci. ISSN 0077-8923

ANNALS OF THE NEW YORK ACADEMY OF SCIENCES
Issue: *Myasthenia Gravis and Related Disorders*

New horizons for congenital myasthenic syndromes

Andrew G. Engel,[1] Xin-Ming Shen,[1] Duygu Selcen,[1] and Steven Sine[2]

[1]Neuromuscular Research Laboratory, Department of Neurology, Mayo Clinic, Rochester, Minnesota. [2]Receptor Biology Laboratory, Department of Physiology and Biomedical Engineering, and Department of Neurology, Mayo Clinic, Rochester, Minnesota

Address for correspondence: Andrew G. Engel, Department of Neurology, Mayo Clinic, 200, Street SW, Rochester, MN 55905. age@mayo.edu

During the past five years an increasing number of patients have been diagnosed with congenital myasthenic syndromes (CMS) and a number of novel syndromes have been recognized and investigated. This presentation focuses on the CMS caused by defects in choline acetyltransferase, novel fast-channel syndromes that hinder isomerization of the acetylcholine receptor from the closed to the open state, the consequences of deleterious mutations in the intermediate filament linker plectin, altered neuromuscular transmission in a centronuclear myopathy, and two recently identified CMS caused by congenital defects in glycosylation.

Keywords: congenital myasthenic syndromes; acetylcholine receptor; fast-channel syndromes; choline acetyltransferase; plectin; centronuclear myopathy; GFPT1; DPAGT1

Introduction

The molecular era of the congenital myasthenic syndromes (CMS) came of age in 1995 with discovery that a highly disabling slow-channel CMS was caused by a gain-of-function point mutation in the second transmembrane domain of the AChR ε subunit. Since then, no fewer than 14 disease genes have been identified, and the tools of molecular genetics empowered the candidate gene approach. Linkage analysis and more recently exome sequencing studies also helped pinpoint disease genes and mutations. Table 1 shows a classification of 350 CMS kinships investigated at the Mayo Clinic to date. The table is still incomplete because in half as many kinships the molecular basis of the CMS remains undefined. This presentation focuses on selected CMS recently investigated in our laboratory.

Choline acetyltransferase (ChAT) deficiency

We have investigated 18 unrelated patients with this CMS. The first five were seen before 2001[1] and 13 others in the past decade; 11 of 13 patients harboring one nonsense and 12 missense mutation were further investigated[2] (Fig. 1A). Abrupt episodes of apnea or severe dyspnea against a variable background of myasthenic symptoms remains a hallmark of the disease. Five patients presented with apnea and with or without other myasthenic symptoms at birth and five had similar presentation during the first five months of life. Three patients never breathed spontaneously: one died and two others are ventilator dependent at 4 and 10 years of age. One patient was born with multiple joint contractures. Eight affected siblings of four patients died in infancy. Pyridostigmine treatment improved but did not remove the symptoms in nine patients and had no effect in four severely affected patients.

To better understand the phenotypic variability of the disease, we determined expression of the recombinant mutants in heterologous cells, analyzed their kinetic properties and thermal stability, and interpreted their functional effects in the context of the atomic structural model of human ChAT at 2.2 Å resolution.[3,4] We examined expression of missense mutants at the protein level by genetically engineering mutant and wild-type *CHAT* cDNAs into Bosc 23 cells and analyzed immunoblots of cell lysates. Eight mutants expressed at significantly lower levels than wild-type, and five of these (W421S, S498P, T553N, p.A557T, p.S572W) expressed at <50% of wild type.

doi: 10.1111/j.1749-6632.2012.06803.x

Table 1. Classification of the Mayo Cohort of CMS patients[a]

	Index cases
Presynaptic defects (6%)	
Choline acetyltransferase deficiency[b]	18
Paucity of synaptic vesicles and reduced quantal release	1
Lambert-Eaton syndrome like	1
Synaptic basal lamina–associated defects (13%)	
Endplate AChE deficiency[b]	45
β2-laminin deficiency[b]	1
Postsynaptic defects (67%)	
Primary kinetic abnormality of AChR (slow- and fast-channel syndromes)[b]	62
Primary AChR deficiency[b]	118
Rapsyn deficiency[b]	51
Plectin deficiency[b]	2
Na-channel myasthenia[b]	1
Defects in endplate development and maintenance (14%)	
DOK7 myasthenia[b]	35
GFPT1 deficiency[b]	11
DAPGT1 deficiency[b]	2
Agrin deficiency[b]	1
CMS with centronuclear myopathy	1
Total (100%)	350

[a]One hundred and twenty-six patients also underwent intercostal muscle biopsies.
[b]Gene defect identified.

To evaluate the kinetic parameters and thermal stability of wild-type and mutant ChAT, we transformed *E. coli* with histidine-tagged *CHAT* cDNAs and purified the enzymes recovered from the bacterial cell lysates on a Ni-NTA column followed by fast protein liquid chromatography. Ten mutations alter one or more rate constants of ChAT activation and hence the catalytic efficiency of the enzyme. Two mutations that introduce a Pro residue into an alpha helix (S498P and S704P) have little effect on enzyme kinetics but compromise the thermal stability of the mutant protein. The most severely affected patients harbored at least one mutation near the active site tunnel (M202R, T553N, and A557T) (Fig. 1B) or the agonist binding site (S572W) (Fig. 1C) of the enzyme and some of these also curtailed enzyme expression.

Novel fast-channel mutations in AChR

Fast-channel CMS are caused by recessive loss-of-function mutations of the AChR. The mutations become pathogenic when accompanied by a low-expressor or null mutation in the second allele or if they occur at homozygosity. The mutations exert their effect by decreasing agonist affinity or by impeding isomerization of the receptor from the closed to the open state.

Homozygous εW55R mutation at the α/ε binding site interface

This mutation was observed in an 8-year-old boy born to consanguineous parents with severe myasthenic symptoms that responded poorly to pyridostigmine.[5] Three similarly affected siblings died in infancy. The mutated Trp55 is one of several negatively charged aromatic residues at the α/ε binding site required to stabilize cationic ACh by electrostatic forces (Fig. 2A–C). Thus replacement of the electron-rich Trp by a cationic Arg was expected to hinder binding of ACh to the α/ε binding site. Single-channel recordings from εW55R-AChR expressed in HEK cells at low ACh concentration (50 nM) revealed that the length of the dominant component of channel opening bursts was reduced to 10% of wild type (Fig. 2E). Analysis of channel openings over a range of ACh concentrations demonstrated that the εW55R mutation reduces apparent agonist affinity at the α/ε binding site by 30-fold and decreases apparent gating efficiency by 75-fold. The mutation also curtails the opening probability of the receptor (P_{open}) over a wide range of ACh concentration (Fig. 2D). In the presence of 1 mM ACh, which corresponds to the estimated peak ACh concentration in the synaptic space after quantal release, the P_{open} of the mutant receptor is only 10% of wild type, which explains the patient's refractoriness to clinically attainable doses of pyridostigmine.

αV188M mutation in the AChR C-loop hinders initiation of channel gating

According to current knowledge, the C-loop alters its conformation during agonist binding. Without agonist, it adopts a range of open conformations that allow the agonist to enter the binding pocket. When the agonist binds, the C-loop moves inward, traps the agonist, and thereby initiates the chain of events that culminate in opening of the ion channel.[6–9]

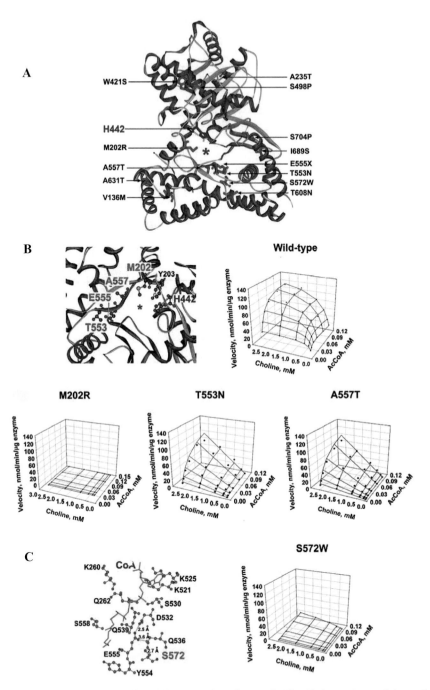

Figure 1. Recently identified mutations in ChAT. (A) Human ChAT showing the identified mutations and the catalytic His442 at the active site. The asterisk indicates the active-site tunnel. (B) Positions of mutated residues in the active site tunnel and kinetic landscapes of wild-type and mutant enzymes. The p.M202R mutant is essentially inactive. T553N and A557T mutants fail to saturate within the indicated range of substrate concentrations. (C) Position of S572 and kinetic landscape of the S572W-ChAT. S572 is close to the AcCoA and choline binding sites. This mutation markedly reduces k_{cat} and K_m for both substrates. (PDB 2FY2). (Reprinted from Ref. 2, by permission.)

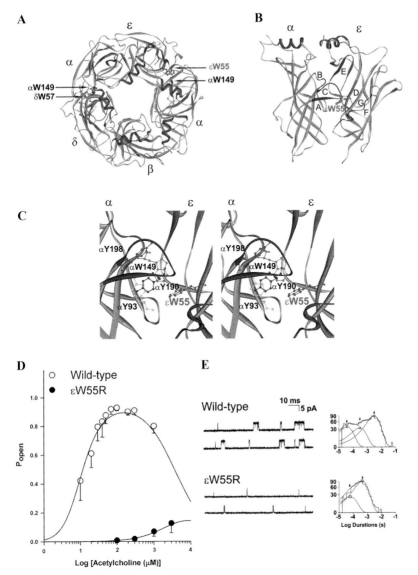

Figure 2. The εW55R mutation at the AChR α/ε binding site. (A) Structural model of extracellular domains of human AChR viewed from the synaptic space, indicating positions of Trp residues at the α/δ and α/ε binding sites. (PDB 1 9B) (B) Side-view of the α and ε subunits showing position of loops E, D, G, and F in the ε subunit, and loops A, B, and C in the α subunit. (C) Stereo view of the binding site showing positions of aromatic residues shrouding the binding pocket. In each panel, the mutated εTrp55 at the α/ε binding site is highlighted in red: based on the crystal structure of the ACh binding protein (PDB 19B) and lysine scanning mutagenesis delineating the structure of the human AChR binding domain. (D) Channel open probability (P_{open}) of ε W55R–AChR, as a function of ACh concentration. Symbols and vertical lines indicate means and standard deviations. Smooth curves are P_{open} predicted by the fitted rate constants. (E) Single-channel currents elicited from HEK cells transfected with wild-type and εW55R-AChR. Left: Representative channel openings elicited by 50 nM ACh. Right: Logarithmically binned burst duration histograms fitted to the sum of exponentials. The arrows indicate mean duration of burst components. (Reprinted from Ref. 5, by permission.)

An αV188M mutation in the C-loop (Fig. 3A) was observed in a 42-year-old woman with severe myasthenic symptoms since birth.[10] She also carries a heteroallelic low-expressor αG74C mutation in the main immunogenic region; hence αV188M determines the phenotype. Light and electron microscopy studies of intercostal muscle endplates (EPs) demonstrated no structural abnormality.

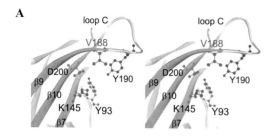

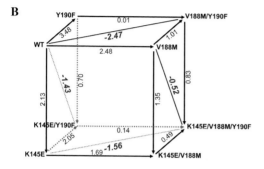

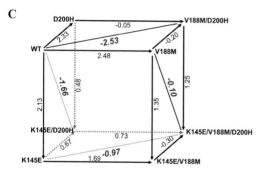

Figure 3. The α_1 AChR subunit binding site and mutant cycle analysis of potentially interacting residues. (A) Stereo view of the binding site at 1.9 Å resolution (PDB 2QC1) shows spatial disposition of the potentially interacting residues. (B) Cubic mutant cycle analysis of energetic interactions between αV188, αY190, and αK145. (C) Cubic mutant cycle analysis of energetic interactions between αV188, αD200, and αK145. In (B) and (C), numbers on arrows show difference in free energy change ($\Delta\Delta$G) between two different AChRs in kcal/mol. The indicated diagonal lines in planes show first-order coupling free energy ($\Delta\Delta$G$_{int}$) for a given pair of mutants, except for the front planes of B and C, where it is $\Delta\Delta$G$_{int}$ = −0.78 kcal/mol, and for the back planes of B and C, where it is $\Delta\Delta$G$_{int}$ = 0.13 and 0.78 kcal/mol, respectively. (Reprinted from Ref. 10, by permission.)

When wild-type and mutant receptors were expressed in HEK cells and their openings monitored by patch-clamp, the length of the predominant burst duration of the mutant receptor was only 20% of the wild type. Detailed kinetic analysis of single channel recordings obtained over a range of ACh concentrations revealed that the most significant effect

of αV188M is a ~70-fold decrease of the apparent channel gating efficiency θ, defined by the ratio of the channel opening rate α to the channel closing rate β. The derived rate constants of activation allowed calculation of P_{open} as a function of ACh concentration. A plot of P_{open} over 3 orders of magnitude of ACh concentrations revealed a marked right shift of P_{open} of the mutant compared to the wild-type receptor. Substitution for Val188 with residues of larger or smaller side-chain volume again reduced the channel opening rate.

To elucidate how αV188M hinders channel opening, we employed thermodynamic mutant cycle analysis[11] to test whether αV188 is energetically coupled to nearby αY190, αD200, and αK145, and whether α these residues contribute jointly to closure of the C-loop after agonist binding (Fig. 3A).[12] The principle of mutant cycle analysis is that the free energy change caused by mutation of residue *A* depends on other residues in the protein. If mutation of a second residue *B* alters the free energy change caused by mutation of *A*, then *A* and *B* are energetically coupled. If mutation of a third residue *C* alters the interactive free energy of the coupling residues *A* and *B*, then *C* also contributes to the interaction between *A* and *B*.

We cast the results of the mutant cycle experiments into two three-dimensional cubic mutant cycles. This analysis revealed that αV188 is strongly coupled with αY190 (Fig. 3B, top face) and also with αD200 (Fig. 3C, top face), but not with αK145 (front faces in Fig. 3B and C). We also found that αK145 contributes to energetic coupling between αV188 and αY190 (Fig. 3B, top and bottom faces) and between αV188 and αD200 (top and bottom faces in Fig. 3C). Further studies revealed that energetic coupling between αK145/αY190 also depends on αV188 (left and right faces in Fig. 3B). Moreover, αV188 also contributes to the energetic coupling between αK145 and αD200 (left and right faces in Fig. 3C). Thus αV188 emerges as a key residue that orchestrates rearrangement of the C-loop during initial coupling of binding to gating.

CMS caused by plectin deficiency

Plectin, encoded by *PLEC*, is a 499–533 kDa dumbbell-shaped intermediate filament cytolinker with multiple isoforms due to exon 1 splice variants. Muscle isoforms link the intermediate filament cytoskeleton to myofibrils, sarcolemma, mitochondria, and nuclear envelope proteins. A skin isoform links epidermal keratin filaments to dermal integrin filaments. The predictable consequences of plectin deficiency in muscle are dislocation of myofiber organelles, gaps in the sarcolemma, and degenerating junctional folds. In skin, plectin deficiency results in epidermolysis bullosa simplex (EBS) due to dermoepidermal disjunction.

The two patients observed by us, respectively, carry a Q2057X and p.R2319X and a shared c.12043dupG mutation[13,14] Both patients had EBS since infancy and later developed a progressive myopathy and myasthenic syndrome refractory to pyridostigmine. Both had a decremental EMG response on repetitive nerve stimulation and half-normal amplitude miniature EP potentials (MEPPs). One patient became motionless at age 37 years and died at age 42. The second patient is severely disabled in her 30s. Morphologic studies of both patients revealed dislocated and degenerating muscle fiber organelles (Fig. 4A–D), and plasma membrane defects (Fig. 4E) resulting in Ca^{2+} overloading of the muscle fibers as in Duchenne dystrophy, and extensive degeneration of the junctional folds (Fig. 4F), all attributable to lack of cytoskeletal support.[14]

CMS in centronuclear myopathy

Centronuclear myopathy (CNM) is a clinically and genetically heterogeneous congenital disorder diagnosed by the presence of central nuclei in the majority of muscle fibers with only few or no necrotic or regenerating fibers. The disease genes identified to date are myotubularin (*MTM1*), dynamin 2 (*DNM2*), amphiphysin 2 (*BIN1*), and skeletal muscle ryanodine receptor (*RYR1*), but several patients diagnosed by pathologic criteria have no identified mutations. Apart from limb weakness, ptosis and ophthalmoparesis often occur in all genetically identified CNM subtypes, and some CNM patients fatigue abnormally. One CNM patient with myasthenic features had a homozygous missense mutation in *BIN1*.[15] Four CNM patients with myasthenic features responding to pyridostigmine with no known mutation were also reported, but EP structure and parameters of neuromuscular transmission were not evaluated.[16]

We investigated an adult CNM patient with myasthenic features.[17] His early motor development was normal but he never ran well. At age 13 years, he had fatigable limb-muscle weakness and mild eyelid ptosis. At age 39 years, he had a 19–35% EMG decrement. He responded well to pyridostigmine. Mutation analysis showed no mutations in currently identified CNM disease genes.

EP studies revealed pre- and postsynaptic abnormalities. Synaptic contacts visualized by the cholinesterase reaction showed multiple EP regions on single fibers suggesting remodeling. Quantitative EM revealed simplified postsynaptic regions, normal nerve terminal size, normal synaptic vesicle density, and mild AChR deficiency. The amplitude of the miniature EP potential (MEPP) was reduced to 60% of normal and its decay time was 1.5-fold prolonged pointing to presence of fetal AChR at the EPs. Quantal release by nerve impulse (*m*) was reduced to 40% of normal due to decreased number of quanta available for release. The decreased MEPP amplitude could be due to a combination of factors: simplification of the postsynaptic region reduces the input resistance of the muscle fiber and hence the MEPP amplitude; the decreased number of AChRs per EP; and presence of immature AChRs at the EP that generate lower amplitude MEEPs than adult AChRs. The decreased quantal release by nerve impulse could be due to decreased synaptic contacts per muscle fiber or to a defect in the synaptic vesicle cycle. Because the cholinesterase reactive synaptic contact areas of the fibers were not appreciably reduced, the decrease in *m* likely signals a defect in the synaptic vesicle cycle.

CMS caused congenital defect in glycosylation

Glycosylation of nascent peptides increases their solubility, folding, assembly, and intracellular transport.[18,19,20] Two enzymes involved in glycosylation, glutamine fructose-6-phosphate transaminase (GFPT1) and dolichol phospate-GlycNac-1-phosphotransferase (DPAGT1), are now known to be associated with CMS. GFPT1 controls the flux of glucose into the hexosamine pathway, and hence the biosynthesis of *N*-acetylglucosamine, a key component of glycosyl residues for *N*- and *O*-linked glycosylation of proteins. DPAGT1 catalyzes the first committed step in the path of *N*-glycosylation.

CMS caused by defects in GFPT1

This CMS was identified in 2011 by Senderek *et al.*[21] by linkage and homozygosity analysis studies of multiplex kinships with limb-girdle CMS

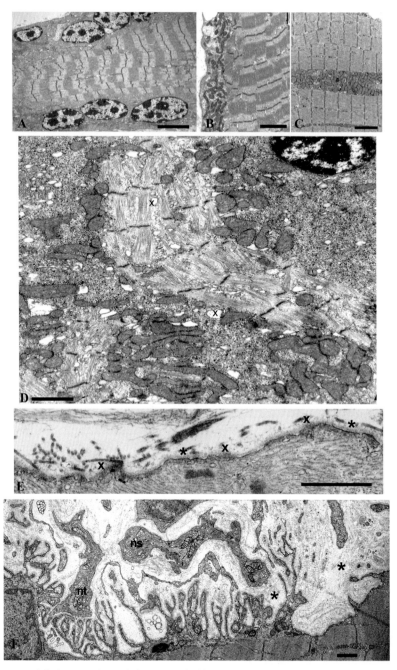

Figure 4. Ultrastructural findings in plectin-deficient muscle fiber. (A) Note subsarcolemmal rows of large nuclei harboring multiple prominent chromatin bodies. (B) and (C) Subsarcolemmal and intrafiber clusters of mitochondria surrounded by fiber regions devoid of mitochondria. (D) Aberrant and disrupted myofibrils surrounded by clusters of mitochondria intermingled with glycogen, ribosomes, and dilated vesicles (x). Note preapoptotic nucleus at upper right. (E) Focal sarcolemma defects due to gaps in the plasma membrane. Where the plasma membrane is absent, the overlying basal lamina is thickened (x). Small vesicles underlie the thickened basal lamina. Asterisks indicate segments of the preserved plasma membrane. (F) Degenerating EP in plectin deficiency. On the left, the postsynaptic region is only partially occupied by the nerve terminal (nt). The center of the panel shows that a nerve sprout (ns) and a nerve terminal are separated by a widened synaptic space from the underlying junctional folds. Many folds are atrophic and degenerating. Streaks of collapsed basal lamina and small globular residues represent remnants of preexisting folds (asterisks). Bars = 4 μm in (A), 3 μm in (B), (C), 1.4 μm in (D), and 1 μm in (E) and (F). (Reprinted from Ref. 14, by permission.)

associated with tubular aggregates in skeletal muscle. GFPT1 is expressed in many tissues and has a long muscle-specific isoform (*GFPTL1*). We investigated 11 CMS patients with GFPT1 deficiency. Ten had a childhood onset, slowly progressive limb-girdle weakness responsive to pyridostigmine. In contrast, one patient did not move *in utero* and was apneic at birth with multiple joint contractures. At the age of 9 years, she requires ventilatory support and gastrostomy feedings and responds poorly to cholinergic agonists. Interestingly, her mother has dermatomyositis and a high titer of AChR antibodies but no clinical myasthenia. The patient never had antibodies against adult AChR, and tests by Angela Vincent detected no antibodies against fetal AChR in the patient or her mother.

Each patient carries two heteroallelic mutations in *GFPT1*. The most severely affected patient harbors a nonsense mutation and a second mutation that causes skipping the muscle specific exon. EM studies revealed small and simple endplates, the MEPP amplitude was reduced in 3 of 5 patients, and quantal release was compromised in the most severe case.

Parameters of neuromuscular transmission were evaluated by microelectrode studies in five patients. In three, the MEPP amplitude was significantly reduced and this was most marked in patient 6. Quantal release by nerve impulse was normal in four patients, but was markedly.

CMS caused by defects in DPAGT1

We recently identified two CMS patients harboring mutations in *DPAGT1*.[22] While our work was in progress, this CMS was reported by Belaya *et al.*[23] One of our patients is a 16-year-old mentally retarded girl with severe generalized CMS since infancy. One similarly affected sibling also has autistic features. The second patient is a 14-year-old girl with mild cognitive deficits and progressive limb-girdle CMS since infancy. Both responded poorly to anti-AChE therapy. Intercostal muscle specimens in both show small tubular aggregates in type 2 fibers, type 1 fiber atrophy, and a vacuolar myopathy with autophagic features. Endplate studies revealed that quantal release, postsynaptic response to acetylcholine quanta, and EP AChR content are reduced to ~50% of normal. EM shows hypoplastic endplates, very small nerve terminals, and poorly differentiated postsynaptic regions. Exome sequencing in each identified two heteroallelic mutations in *DPAGT1*. Immunoblots of muscle extracts demonstrated reduced glycosylation of proteins. We hypothesize that hypoglycosylation of synapse-specific proteins causes defects in motor as well as central synapses.

Acknowledgments

Work done in our laboratories was supported by Award NS6277 (A.G.E.) and NS31744 (S.S.) from the National Institutes of Neurological Disorders and Stroke and a research grant from the Muscular Dystrophy Association (A.G.E).

Conflicts of interest

The authors declare no conflicts of interest.

References

1. Ohno, K., A. Tsujino, X.M. Shen, *et al.* 2001. Choline acetyltransferase mutations cause myasthenic syndrome associated with episodic apnea in humans. *Proc. Natl. Acad. Sci. USA* **98:** 2017–2022.
2. Shen, X.-M., T.O. Crawford, J. Brengman, *et al.* 2011. Functional consequences and structural interpretation of mutations in human choline acetyltransferase. *Hum. Mutat.* **32:** 1259–1267.
3. Kim, A.R., T. Dobransky, R.J. Rylett & B.H. Shilton 2005. Surface-entropy reduction used in the crystallization of human choline acetyltransferase. *Acta Crystallogr.* **Sect. D 61**: 1306–1310.
4. Kim, A.-R., R.J. Rylett & B.H. Shilton 2006. Substrate binding and catalytic mechanism of human choline acetyltransferase. *Biochemistry* **45:** 14621–14631.
5. Engel, A.G., J. Brengman, S. Edvardson, *et al.* 2011. Highly fatal fast-channel congenital syndrome caused by AChR ε subunit mutation at the agonist binding site. *Neurology* **79:** 449–454.
6. Celie, P.H., S.E. van Rossum-Fikkert, W.J. van Dijk, *et al.* 2004. Nicotine and carbamycholine binding to nicotinic acetylcholine receptors as studied in AChBP crystal structures. *Neuron* **41:** 907–914.
7. Cheng, X., H. Wang, B. Grant, *et al.* 2006. Targeted molecular dynamics study of C-loop closure and channel gating in nicotinic receptors. *PLOS Comput. Biol.* **2:** 1173–1184; e134.
8. Wang, H.-L., R. Toghraee, D. Papke, *et al.* 2009. Single-channel current through nicotinic receptor produced by closure of binding C-loop. *Biophys. J.* **96:** 3582–3590.
9. Li, S.X., S. Huang, N. Bren, *et al.* 2011. Ligand-binding domain of an α7-nicotinic receptor chimera and its complex with agonist. *Nat. Neurosci.* **14:** 1253–1259.
10. Shen, X.-M., J. Brengman, S.M. Sine & A.G. Engel. 2012. Myasthenic syndrome AChRα C-loop mutant disrupts initiation of channel gating. *J. Clin. Invest.* **122:** 2613–2621.
11. Horovitz, A. & A. Fersht. 1990. Strategy for analyzing the cooperativity of intramolecular interactions in peptides and proteins. *J. Mol. Biol.* **214:** 613–617.

12. Mukhtasimova, N., C. Free & S.M. Sine. 2005. Initial coupling of binding to gating mediated by conserved residues in muscle nicotinic receptor. *J. Gen. Physiol.* **126:** 23–39.

13. Banwell, B.L., J. Russel, T. Fukudome, *et al.* 1999. Myopathy, myasthenic syndrome, and epidermolysis bullosa simplex due to plectin deficiency. *J. Neuropathol. Exp. Neurol.* **58:** 832–846.

14. Selcen, D., V.C. Juel, L.D. Hobson-Webb, *et al.* 2011. Myasthenic syndrome caused by plectinopathy. *Neurology* **76:** 327–336.

15. Claeys, K.G., T. Maisonobe, J. Bohm, *et al.* 2010. Phenotype of a patient with recessive centronuclear myopathy and a novel BIN1 mutation. *Neurology* **74:** 519–521.

16. Robb, S.A., C.A. Sewry, J.J. Dowling, *et al.* 2011. Impaired neuromuscular transmission and response to aceyl-cholinesterase inhibitors in centronuclear myopathy. *Neuromuscul. Disord.* **21:** 379–386.

17. Liewluck, T., X.-M. Shen, M. Milone & A.G. Engel. 2011. Endplate structure and parameters of neuromuscular transmission in sporadic centronuclear myopathy associated with myasthenia. *Neuromuscul. Disord.* **21:** 387–395.

18. Haeuptle, M.A. & T. Hennet. 2009. Congenital disorders of glycosylation: an update on defects affecting the biosynthesis of dolichol-linked oligosaccharides. *Hum. Mutat.* **30:** 1628–1641.

19. Freeze, H.H. & V. Sharma. 2010. Metabolic manipulation of glycosylation disorders in humans and animal models. *Semin. Cell Dev. Biol.* **21:** 655–662.

20. Freeze, H.H, E.A. Eklund, B.G. Ng & M.C. Patterson. 2012. Neurology of inherited glycosylation disordrs. *Lancet Neurol.* **11:** 453–466.

21. Senderek, J., J.S. Muller, M. Dusl, *et al.* 2011. Hexosamine biosynthetic pathway mutations cause neuromuscular transmission defect. *Am. J. Hum. Genet.* **88:** 162–172.

22. Selcen, D., X.-M. Shen, Y. Li, *et al.* 2012. Congenital myasthenic syndrome, autophagic myopathy, and cognitive dysfunction caused by mutaions in *DPAGT1*. *Ann. Neurol.* (Abstract). In press.

23. Belaya, K., S. Finlayson, C. Slater, *et al.* 2012. Mutations in DPAGT1 cause a limb-girdle congenital myasthenic syndrome with tubular aggregates. *Am. J. Hum. Genet.* **91:** 1–9.

Ann. N.Y. Acad. Sci. ISSN 0077-8923

ANNALS OF THE NEW YORK ACADEMY OF SCIENCES
Issue: *Myasthenia Gravis and Related Disorders*

Synaptic dysfunction in congenital myasthenic syndromes

David Beeson

Weatherall Institute of Molecular Medicine, The John Radcliffe Hospital, Oxford OX3 9DS, United Kingdom

Address for correspondence: David Beeson, Weatherall Institute of Molecular Medicine, The John Radcliffe Hospital, Oxford OX3 9DS, United Kingdom. David.Beeson@ndcn.ox.ac.uk

Congenital myasthenic syndromes (CMS) are hereditary disorders of neuromuscular transmission characterized by fatigable muscle weakness. The number of cases recognized is increasing with improved diagnosis. To date we have identified over 300 different mutations present in over 350 unrelated kinships. The underlying genetic defects are diverse, involving a series of different genes with a variety of different phenotypes. The type of treatment and its effectiveness will depend on the underlying pathogenic mechanism. We aim to define the molecular mechanism for each mutation identified and feed this information back to the clinic as a basis to tailor patient treatment. Here, we describe some of the methods that can be used to define if a DNA sequence variant is pathogenic with reference to variants in *DOK7*. We highlight a new mechanism for disruption of AChR function, where a mutation in the AChR ε-subunit gene causes reduced ion channel conductance and discuss new methods for identifying gene mutations. The study of these disorders is proving highly informative for understanding the diverse molecular mechanisms that can underlie synaptic dysfunction.

Keywords: congenital myasthenic syndrome; functional diagnostics; DOK7; low conductance mutation, DPAGT1

Introduction

The congenital myasthenic syndromes (CMS) are a heterogeneous group of disorders caused by mutations in a series of different genes that affect neuromuscular transmission. To date at least 15 different genes have been associated with these disorders.[1,2] The base phenotype of fatigable muscle weakness is shared among syndromes, and although there may be phenotypic clues, predicting which genes are defective from clinical examination is often challenging. Most cases can at least be partially treated, and in many cases treatment leads to a profound benefit in the quality of life of the patient.[3] However, appropriate treatment depends upon the underlying molecular mechanism. For instance, in the slow channel syndrome, where there is an excitotoxic effect, the current medical treatment is based on the use of channel blockers that fasten the kinetics of the acetylcholine receptor (AChR) ion channel without inhibiting signal transmission, whereas in fast channel syndromes, treatment strategies are based on increasing the availability of the neurotransmitter acetylcholine. If the genetic basis and the underlying molecular mechanism for a congenital myasthenic syndrome can be determined, then treatment can be tailored to the individual patient. In many centers, targeted genetic screening is now the main method used for determining which congenital myasthenic syndrome the patient harbors.[2] In this approach phenotypic clues gathered from clinical examination, such as eye muscle involvement, patterns of muscle weakness, and occurrence of apneic attacks and joint contractures, and neurophysiology results are fed into an algorithm to determine the order in which genes are screened for the presence of mutations. This method has proved extremely effective, and at the Oxford, UK genetics service we have identified mutations in over 350 kinships (Table 1). However, with the advent of next-generation sequencing techniques, it is probable that over the next five years bioinformatics applied to whole genome and whole exome sequence data will play a new and critical role in genetic diagnosis. Although there are several more common mutations likely associated with founder

doi: 10.1111/nyas.12000

Table 1. Numbers of the more common congenital myasthenic syndromes analyzed in Oxford, classified by genetic screening and functional analysis of mutations

Syndrome	Kinships
AChR deficiency (*CHRNE*)	146
AChR deficiency (*RAPSN*)	73
CMS with proximal weakness (*DOK7*)	68
Slow channel (*CHRNA/B/D/E*)	25
Fast channel (*CHRNA/D/E*)	15
AChE deficiency (*COLQ*)	20
Presynaptic (*CHAT*)	8

effects, such as the c.1267delG[4] or 1293[5] mutation in *CHRNE* or the p.Asp88Lys missense mutation in *RAPSN*,[6] most CMS-associated genes have multiple "private" mutations, many of which are missense mutations. Although several software programs are available for predicting whether a sequence variant is likely to be pathogenic, more often than not proof of pathogenicity is best established through functional analysis of the variant protein in cell culture systems. We highlight some of the functional assays that we routinely use to determine pathogenicity of genetic variants that we encounter when screening DNA for CMS.

DOK7 mutations

As stated in the chapter on the clinical features of *DOK7* CMS, DOK7 is an adaptor protein that binds to MuSK and amplifies the signaling pathway that is largely responsible both for neuromuscular junction synapse formation and then subsequently for maintaining the synaptic structure.[7] Within the human population the *DOK7* gene shows a high degree of variability and screening for mutations reveals numerous sequence variants. Some variants can be eliminated by reference to human variation databases such as dbSNP,[8] or by segregation analysis, but in many cases the variants are rare and other family members are not available for analysis. When myoblasts from C2C12 mouse muscle cell line are differentiated to form myotubes in culture, clusters of acetylcholine receptors (AChR) can be induced to form on the myotube cell surface by the addition of neural agrin.[9] The agrin interacts with LRP4[10,11] to stimulate MuSK that, in turn, induces the aggregation of AChR into clusters

that can be visualized under the microscope with labeled α-bungarotoxin (Fig. 1A and B). Overexpression of DOK7 in C2C12 myotubes has the remarkable property of inducing AChR clusters in the absence of Agrin.[7] Mutations identified in DOK7 CMS have been shown to impair the efficiency of the induced AChR clustering in C2C12 myotubes,[12] and it is possible to use this model system to determine pathogenicity of DOK7 variants detected in gene screens.[13] A key feature for this system is to ensure a majority of the C2C12 myoblasts are transfected with *DOK7* or the *DOK7* mutant expression constructs before differentiation into myotubes. To ensure the majority of cells express the mutant, a retroviral infection/expression system may be used. Once the myotubes infected with the DOK7 expression construct are formed, the AChR clusters can be visualized following incubation either with fluorescence-labeled α-bungarotoxin or anti-AChR antibodies and pathogenicity determined through a reduction in the number and complexity of the clusters formed. Following screening of possible DOK7 CMS cases, use of this system, in combination with standard molecular genetic techniques, enabled 34 different pathogenic mutations to be identified in 72 patients, and 27 rare variants to be classified as nonpathogenic.[13] Mutation 1124_1127dupTGCC is a common mutation found in over half of reported DOK7 CMS patients. There are several other incidences of truncations in the large 3′ exon of *DOK7* where the properties of the DOK7 protein required for binding MuSK are retained, but an additional though not crucial function in the C-terminus region is lost. Whereas previously described DOK7 CMS cases have a least one allele with a mutation in the last 3′ exon of the gene that encodes a large C-terminal region of the protein,[14–18] it was possible to show that cases occur where mutations in both alleles are present toward the N-terminal region of the protein that contains the pleckstrin homology and phosphotyrosine binding domains. However, even using these techniques to define the nature of the DOK7 variants a few additional cases are found in which only one pathogenic mutation is identified in the coding sequence. Potentially further mutations can be identified at the RNA/protein level through analysis of RNA from patient muscle biopsy,[16] but the location of the mutations that cause altered RNA splicing or expression may only become identifiable when whole genome sequencing is available.

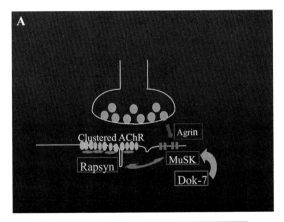

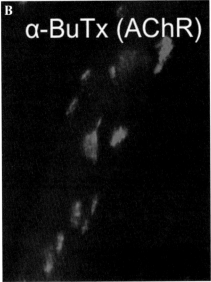

Figure 1. (A) Diagrammatic representation of the Agrin–MuSK–Rapsyn AChR clustering pathway. (B) AChR clusters formed on a C2C12 myotube following incubation with soluble Agrin.

Identification of a large number of mutations in *DOK7,* and their differing effects on the number and complexity of AChR clusters, provides a pool of information that can potentially be used in investigation of the signaling pathway from MuSK activation to the Rapsyn-associated AChR cluster formation that is still largely undetermined.

AGRN, MUSK, and RAPSN mutations

Similar methodologies using cultured muscle cells can be used to analyze the effects of sequence variants identified in genes that encode other key proteins in the AChR clustering pathway. Mutations in

AGRN and *MUSK* are rare, but mutations are more frequently found in *RAPSN.*[2] Other factors such as expression levels may be involved in affecting the function of the respective protein, but analyzing the effect of a mutation on AChR clustering in cultured cells is useful for assessing pathogenicity. For mutations in *MUSK* and *RAPSN* it is helpful to have available muscle cells lines that do not express endogenous MuSK or Rapsyn, whereas for mutations in *AGRN* it is possible to synthesize the mutant protein, add it to differentiated C2C12 myotubes, and to compare AChR clustering to that seen with expressed wild-type agrin.[17] As stated, mutations in *AGRN* and *MUSK* are rare, but this methodology can be used to determine pathogenicity for mutation in *RAPSN* where there are a considerable number of mutations and also nonpathogenic sequence variants.

AChR mutations

During evolution the genes that encode the muscle AChR subunit have been highly conserved. However, screening considerable numbers of potential CMS patients reveals a surprising number of rare variants within the human population. Mutations of the AChR give rise to several different forms of CMS, which include AChR deficiency syndromes, slow channel syndrome, and the fast channel syndrome.[1,2] When cDNAs encoding the four AChR subunits are introduced into HEK 293 cells they express assembled AChR on the cell surface. In patch clamp electrophysiological recordings of single AChR channels the kinetic properties of the assembled AChR resemble those observed *in vivo* from human muscle biopsies.[19] Analysis of the single channel recordings will reveal if a mutation prolongs channel burst duration, abbreviates burst duration, or has no effect. Using these techniques, a standard procedure for analyzing AChR sequence variants is *in vitro* mutagenesis of the respective cDNA, expression of the mutant cDNA in HEK 293, followed by binding of [^{125}I]α-bungarotoxin to the surface of the HEK 293 cells. Rarely, mutations causing AChR deficiency are located in the α, β, or δ subunits, and these can be readily picked up in cell-surface [^{125}I]α-bungarotoxin binding experiments. However, α, β, and δ subunits can combine in the absence of the ε subunit to generate surface [^{125}I]α-bungarotoxin binding, and therefore if the mutation is in *CHRNE* (ε-subunit), levels of expression of the mutant AChR can be determined by immunopre-cipitation of the AChR-[^{125}I]α-bungarotoxin com-plex with an AChRε subunit-specific antibody, which will only detect AChR pentamers harbor-ing the ε subunit. This assay has proved effec-tive in determining if the primary pathogenic mechanism is due to endplate AChR deficiency. Mutations in *CHRNE* causing endplate AChR defi-ciency are the most common cause of CMS (Table 1). If, however, levels of surface expression of the variant AChR are comparable to wild-type AChR, then the variant subunit may be nonpathogenic or have altered channel kinetics, potentially resulting in either a slow channel syndrome or a fast chan-nel syndrome. Single channel patch clamp analysis of the HEK 293 cell-expressed AChR is required to determine either prolonged or shortened chan-nel activations indicative of respective slow chan-nel or fast channel syndromes. In a recent report, a patient was found to have heteroallelic muta-tions in *CHRNE* (p.εP282R and p.εF266del).[20] Mutated p.εP282R showed reduced surface AChR

expression in HEK 293 cells, whereas, surprisingly, p.εF266del expressed well. Thus, it is the proper-ties of p.εF266del that determines the phenotype of the patient. When single channel patch clamp was performed on AChR harboring p.εF266del, the burst duration of the channel activations did not differ significantly from wild-type AChR. How-ever, analysis of the current amplitudes at differing holding potentials demonstrates that this mutation causes a reduced flow of ions through the channel, and thus will impair the depolarization at the end-plate required to activate the voltage-gated sodium channels.

Thus, a novel molecular mechanism has been identified for impaired function of the AChR ion channel (Fig. 2). This mechanism for ion chan-nel dysfunction has long been postulated but it has taken until now to identify a case. The phenotypic features of patients with reduced ion channel con-ductance are likely to share some similarities with the fast channel syndrome,[21] in that both cause a loss of function and require a mutation on the

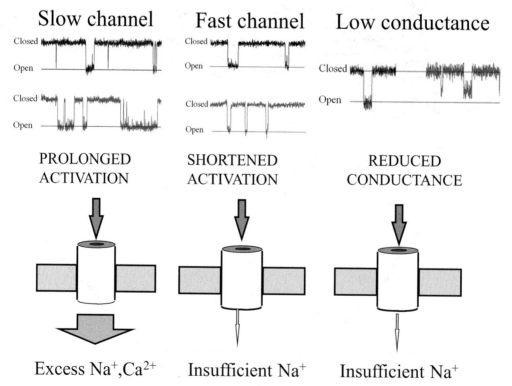

Figure 2. Illustration of the pathogenic mechanisms of disorders of the AChR ion channel. Top panels illustrate patch clamp single AChR channel recording traces: black traces, wild-type channels; red traces, mutant channels. Lower panels illustrate the consequence of altered ion channel function.

second allele to unmask the impaired properties of the ion channel caused by these mutations.

Advent of next-generation sequencing

Methodologies used to identify the gene associated with CMS have relied on a knowledge of key molecules that participate in transmission of signal across the neuromuscular junction or that govern the synaptic structure to provide candidate genes for screening.[1] Alternatively, linkage analysis, if suitable families are available, can be used to define genetic regions that can then be used to home in on further candidate genes.[22] These methodologies have proven fruitful, but there still remain cases in which mutations are yet to be identified. The advent of next-generation sequencing, either exome sequencing or whole-genome sequencing, provides an opportunity to identify the genetic cause in these remaining disorders. Stratification of the phenotype is helpful and has been used to identify mutations

in *DPAGT1*.[22] However, with the mass of data now being gathered from the sequencing of many human genomes, it is potentially possible to identify the mutations in a new gene in a single individual. It is of note that the two most recently identified genes associated with CMS, *GFPT1*[22] and *DPAGT1*,[23] are ubiquitously expressed and thus are not obvious candidates for mutations to cause neuromuscular junction disorders. The next few years should prove fruitful in identifying additional CMS-associated mutations in new genes. These will require additional functional assays to be established in order to determine pathogenicity of rare variants that will inevitably be found.

Treatment of the congenital myasthenic syndromes

A primary reason for functional studies of mutations is to establish the pathogenic mechanism and thereby provide a rational basis for therapy. For

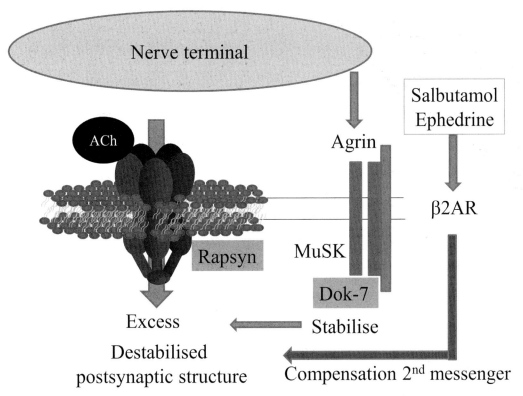

Figure 3. A potential simple model for the action of β2-adrenergic receptor agonists in treatment of selected congenital myasthenic syndromes. Activation of the MuSK-DOK7 pathway initiates a kinase pathway that controls clustering and synapse integrity. Loss of synaptic function is likely to occur if this pathway is impaired. It is possible that activation of second messenger pathways in the vicinity of the motor endplates can partially compensate for impaired MuSK signaling.

example, in the slow channel syndrome the aim would be to block excess cation entry through the AChR at the endplate via drugs that block the channel when in the open state, such as fluoxetine; whereas for a fast channel syndrome one would aim to enhance the postsynaptic signal either through anticholinesterase medication or increased neurotransmitter release via blocking voltage gated potassium cannels with 3,4-diaminopyridine. However, a key advance in the treatment of the CMS in recent years has been the targeted use of the β2-adrenergic receptor agonists ephedrine and salbutamol/albuterol. Following identification of mutations in *DOK7* as a cause of CMS,[12] it became clear that this set of patients gain remarkable benefit from treatment with either ephedrine or salbutamol.[24–27] It is noteworthy that the effect is not immediate but a gradual improvement is experienced over a period of months until the beneficial effects plateau, usually between six months and a year from initiation.[24] Although the effects of these drugs are probably most dramatic in DOK7 CMS there are also several reports of their beneficial effects in other CMS, such as patients with mutations in *COLQ*[28] or even some cases of AChR deficiency.[29] It would appear that the β2-agonists are likely providing compensation through second messenger pathways to help alleviate destabilization of the endplate structures caused by mutations of endplate proteins. A simple diagrammatic model for this is shown in Figure 3. A challenge for the future will be to understand the detail for exactly how these drugs have their effects at the endplate region of muscle. This, in turn, may help point to new drugs and enable further optimization of treatments for congenital myasthenic syndromes.

Conflicts of interest

The author declares no conflicts of interest.

References

1. Engel, A.G. 2012. Current status of the congenital myasthenic syndromes. *Neuromuscul. Disord.* **22:** 99–111
2. Chaouch, A., D. Beeson, D. Hantaï & H. Lochmüller 2012. 186th ENMC international workshop: congenital myasthenic syndromes 24–26 June 2011, Naarden, The Netherlands. *Neuromuscul. Disord.* **22:** 566–576
3. Engel, A.G. 2007. The therapy of congenital myasthenic syndromes. *Neurotherapeutics* **4:** 252–257.
4. Abicht, A. *et al.* 1999. A common mutation (epsilon1267delG) in congenital myasthenic patients of Gypsy ethnic origin. *Neurology* **53:** 1564–1569.
5. Richard, P. *et al.* 2008. The CHRNE 1293insG founder mutation is a frequent cause of congenital myasthenia in North Africa. *Neurology* **71:** 1967–1972.
6. Müller, J.S. *et al.* 2004. The congenital myasthenic syndrome mutation RAPSN N88K derives from an ancient Indo-European founder. *J. Med. Genet.* **41:** e104.
7. Okada, K. *et al.* 2006. The muscle protein Dok-7 is essential for neuromuscular synaptogenesis. *Science* **312:** 1802–1805.
8. Sherry, S.T. *et al.* 2001. dbSNP: the NCBI database of genetic variation. *Nucleic Acids Res.* **29:** 308–311.
9. Sanes, J.R. & J.W. Lichtman. 2001. Induction, assembly, maturation and maintenance of a postsynaptic apparatus. *Nat. Rev. Neurosci.* **2:** 791–805.
10. Zhang, B. *et al.* 2008. LRP4serves as a coreceptor of agrin. *Neuron* **60:** 285–297.
11. Kim, N. *et al.* 2008. Lrp4 is a receptor for Agrin and forms a complex with MuSK. *Cell* **135:** 334–342.
12. Beeson, D. *et al.* 2006. Dok-7 mutations underlie a neuromuscular junction synaptopathy. *Science* **313:** 1975–1978.
13. Cossins, J. *et al.* 2012. The spectrum of mutations that underlie the neuromuscular junction synaptopathy in DOK7 congenital myasthenic syndrome. *Hum. Mol. Genet.* **21:** 3765–3775.
14. Müller, J.S. *et al.* 2007. Phenotypical spectrum of DOK7 mutations in congenital myasthenic syndromes. *Brain* **130:** 1497–1506.
15. Palace *et al.* 2007. Clinical features of the DOK7 neuromuscular junction synaptopathy. *Brain* **130:** 1507–1515.
16. Selcen, D. *et al.* 2008. Dok-7 myasthenia: phenotypic and molecular genetic studies in 16 patients. *Ann. Neurol.* **64:** 71–87.
17. Maselli, R.A. *et al.* 2012. LG2 agrin mutation causing severe congenital myasthenic syndrome mimics functional characteristics of non-neural (z-) agrin. *Hum. Genet.* **131:** 1123–1135
18. Ammar, A.B. *et al.* 2010. Phenotype genotype analysis in 15 patients presenting a congenital myasthenic syndrome due to mutations in DOK7. *J. Neurol.* **257:** 754–766.
19. Ohno, K. *et al.* 1995. Congenital myasthenic syndrome caused by prolonged acetylcholine receptor channel openings due to a mutation in the M2 domain of the epsilon subunit. *Proc. Natl. Acad. Sci. USA* **92:** 758–762.
20. Webster, R. *et al.* 2012. A novel congenital myasthenic syndrome due to decreased acetylcholine receptor ion-channel conductance. *Brain* **135:** 1070–1080.
21. Palace, J. *et al.* 2012. Clinical features in a series of fast channel congenital myasthenia syndrome. *Neuromuscul. Disord.* **22:** 112–117.
22. Senderek, J. *et al.* 2011. Hexosamine biosynthetic pathway mutations cause neuromuscular transmission defect. *Am. J. Hum. Genet.* **88:** 162–172.
23. Belaya, K. *et al.* 2012. Mutations in DPAGT1 cause a limb-girdle congenital myasthenic syndrome with tubular aggregates. *Am. J. Hum. Genet.* **91,** 193–201.
24. Lashley, D., J. Palace, S. Jayawant, *et al.* 2010. Ephedrine treatment in congenital myasthenic syndrome due to mutations in DOK7. *Neurology* **74:** 1517–1523.

25. Schara, U. *et al*. 2009. Ephedrine therapy in eight patients with congenital myasthenic syndrome due to DOK7 mutations. *Neuromuscul. Disord.* **19:** 828–832.

26. Liewluck, T., D. Selcen & A.G. Engel 2011. Beneficial effects of albuterol in congenital endplate acetylcholinesterase deficiency and Dok-7 myasthenia. *Muscle Nerve* **44:** 789–794.

27. Burke, G. *et al*. 2011. Salbutamol treatment in children with DOK7 congenital myasthenic syndrome. *Eur. J. Paed. Neurol.* **15**(Suppl 1): 2 Abstract.

28. Chan, S.H., V.C. Wong & A.G. Engel. 2012. Neuromuscular junction acetylcholinesterase deficiency responsive to albuterol. *Pediatr. Neurol.* **47:** 137–140.

29. Sadeh, M., X.M. Shen & A.G. Engel. 2011. Beneficial effect of albuterol in congenital myasthenic syndrome with epsilon-subunit mutations. *Muscle Nerve* **44:** 289–291.

Ann. N.Y. Acad. Sci. ISSN 0077-8923

ANNALS OF THE NEW YORK ACADEMY OF SCIENCES
Issue: *Myasthenia Gravis and Related Disorders*

SOX1 antibodies in Lambert–Eaton myasthenic syndrome and screening for small cell lung carcinoma

Alexander F. Lipka,[1] Jan J.G.M. Verschuuren,[1] and Maarten J. Titulaer[1,2]

[1]Department of Neurology, Leiden University Medical Center, Leiden, the Netherlands. [2]Department of Neuroimmunology, Institut d'Investigació Biomèdica August Pi I Sunyer (IDIBAPS), Hospital Clinic, University of Barcelona, Barcelona, Spain

Address for correspondence: Maarten J. Titulaer, MD, PhD, Department of Neuroimmunology, Institut d'Investigació Biomèdica August Pi I Sunyer (IDIBAPS) Hospital Clinic, University of Barcelona, Casanova, 143; Floor 5, Lab 503, Department 2, Barcelona, 08036, Spain. m.j.titulaer@lumc.nl

Lambert–Eaton myasthenic syndrome (LEMS) is an autoimmune disorder of the neuromuscular synapse. About half of LEMS patients have an associated small cell lung carcinoma (SCLC), which is usually detected after diagnosis of LEMS. This short review summarizes clinical and serological markers shown to predict the presence of SCLC in LEMS patients. SOX1 antibodies are a specific marker for SCLC-LEMS but they are also found in SCLC patients without paraneoplastic neurological syndromes. No relation to any clinical characteristic or survival effect has been found for SOX1-positive patients. Several clinical markers also discriminate between SCLC-LEMS and nontumor LEMS. Detailed analysis of these clinical and demographic characteristics from two independent patient cohorts has led to development of the DELTA-P score. This prediction model has provided for a simple clinical tool to indicate the presence of SCLC early in the course of the disease. The DELTA-P score can be used to guide tumor screening in individual patients.

Keywords: Lambert–Eaton myasthenic syndrome; small cell lung cancer; SOX antibodies; screening

Introduction

Lambert–Eaton myasthenic syndrome (LEMS) is an autoimmune disorder of the neuromuscular junction characterized by proximal muscle weakness, loss of tendon reflexes, and autonomic dysfunction.[1,2] It can occur at all ages and affects both men and women. LEMS is caused by pathogenic antibodies against the presynaptic P/Q-type voltage-gated calcium channel (VGCC), found in most patients.[3] In about 50–60% of patients, small cell lung cancer (SCLC) is detected.[1,4,5] Diagnosis of LEMS usually precedes diagnosis of SCLC, thus prompting vigorous tumor screening.[6,7] Until recently, the efficiency of screening modalities has been under discussion and optimal screening methods for associated lung cancer were based on expert opinion. Several factors have been shown to predict the presence of SCLC, though none of these markers was accurate enough to guide screening individually.

This short review focuses on clinical and serological markers to discriminate between SCLC-related LEMS (SCLC-LEMS) and nontumor LEMS (NT-LEMS). The discovery of SOX1 antibodies in LEMS has both increased our understanding of the immunopathophysiology of paraneoplastic LEMS and aided in discriminating between SCLC-LEMS and NT-LEMS. However, the most relevant discrimination between these two groups can accurately be derived from clinical markers using the DELTA-P score.[8]

Pathophysiology

Antibodies against P/Q type VGCC are presumed to be pathogenic in most LEMS patients. This antigen is present both in SCLC and the presynaptic part of the neuromuscular junction.[9] A pathogenic role for these antibodies is supported by passive transfer and mouse model studies.[10–12] Although both paraneoplastic and NT-LEMS are positive for VGCC antibodies in about 90% of patients, it is likely that part of the initial immunopathophysiologal pathway differs between the tumor and nontumor form.[3,4] In SCLC-LEMS, the presence of VGCC on SCLC cells

doi: 10.1111/j.1749-6632.2012.06772.x
Ann. N.Y. Acad. Sci. 1275 (2012) 70–77 © 2012 New York Academy of Sciences.

elicits an immune response resulting in the production of VGCC antibodies.

In LEMS patients without associated tumor the mechanism for triggering the autoimmune response remains unknown. Several demographic and genetic characteristics suggest that these patients are more susceptible to developing autoimmune diseases. An increased frequency of other autoimmune diseases has been shown in both patients and their family in NT-LEMS patients.[13] A genetic association is described with the HLA B8-DR3 haplotype.[5,14] This HLA 8.1 ancestral haplotype is most closely associated with young female patients, both in NT-LEMS and early onset myasthenia gravis, and is linked to various other autoimmune diseases.[14–16]

Tumor association

About 50–60% of LEMS patients have an associated tumor, almost invariably an SCLC. SCLC accounts for approximately 13–16% of pulmonary tumors and is aggressive, with a median survival in patients of only 10 months.[17,18] It is strongly related to smoking and has neuroendocrine characteristics, which partly explains the relatively frequent cooccurrence of paraneoplastic neurological syndromes (PNSs).[2] Sporadic cases with non-SCLC, prostate carcinoma, thymoma, and lymphoproliferative disorders have been described.[1,4,6] It is difficult to prove a relation between rare cases of LEMS and highly prevalent tumors. In individual cases the likelihood of a causal relationship between tumor and the occurrence of LEMS can be supported by demonstrating neuroendocrine characteristics of the tumor.[19]

An impressive prolonged survival has been observed in patients with SCLC and LEMS, which may be due to the fact that antibodies target an extracellular accessible antigen (VGCC) on SCLC cells, and activate complement or antibody-mediated cytotoxicity. Alternatively, a T cell–mediated cytotoxic immune response against SCLC tumor cells expressing VGCC or other onconeural antigens could be responsible for the beneficial antitumor immune response. Three studies report a significantly prolonged median survival of 17, 20, and 24 months in SCLC-LEMS patients compared to 10 months in SCLC patients without this paraneoplastic disease.[20–22] Three-year survival is 33% versus 2%, respectively.[5] This is partly explained by lead time bias,

indicating LEMS diagnosis leads to earlier detection of the tumor and a "longer survival," even in the absence of an actual effect on survival. The advantage is that the SCLC is subsequently treated earlier and more frequently in a limited stage, which adds to a real positive effect on survival. In addition, an ongoing antitumor immune response retarding tumor growth is probably also present.

Small cell lung carcinoma–associated antibodies and pareneoplastic neurological symptoms

SCLC is a highly immunogenic tumor, frequently eliciting antibodies against tumor antigens.[23] Many of the SCLC-associated antigens are also present in the nervous system, due to the neuroendocrine origin of SCLC. Immune tolerance for these central nervous system antigens is often low, thereby lowering the threshold to involve these antigens in an autoimmune disease.[24–26] Many of these onconeural antibodies have been described in SCLC along with specific PNSs such as the anti-Hu antibody associated with sensory neuronopathy or the anti-CV2 antibody associated with encephalomyelitis.[27] Although only a small proportion of SCLC patients develop PNS, these onconeural antibodies can be found in many more tumor patients without neurological symptoms. For example, VGCC antibodies can be detected in up to 5–8% of SCLC patients without corresponding symptoms in a majority of patients.[28,29] Hu antibodies are detected even more frequently in 13–25% of SCLC patients, whereas less than 1% develop the corresponding paraneoplastic encephalomyelitis or sensory neuropathy.[28,30,31] Some onconeural antibodies in SCLC are not associated with any clinical characteristic or syndrome, but can still be of use for studying the antitumor immune response or serve as a marker for the presence of an SCLC.[32]

SOX proteins

In recent years, a new marker associated with paraneoplastic neurological disease has been described.[33] In a search for new onconeural antibodies, Graus *et al.* detected immunoreactivity to the Bergmann glia of the Purkinje cell layer of rat cerebellum, defined as antiglial nuclear antibody (AGNA).[33] Screening of a fetal brain laboratory identified the antigen as SOX1, which additionally led to improved assays to detect these antibodies.[34] The subsequent detection of SOX1 and related SOX proteins specifically in the Purkinje cell layer of adult human cerebellum supported these findings.[35]

The SOX1 protein is part of a SRY-like high-mobility group superfamily of developmental transcription factors. This protein is part of the SOXB1 group along with SOX2 and SOX3, which share common functions and are expressed in an overlapping manner.[36] These proteins are thought to prevent neural differentiation in progenitor cells and are mainly expressed in the developing nervous system and downregulated in adults. SOX proteins also play a role in airway epithelial differentiation and are shown to be present in SCLC.[32,37] Serological analysis of the humoral immune response in SCLC patients isolated SOX1 and SOX2 as important immunogenic targets.[32] In subsequent studies, SOX1 antibodies were shown to be present in 22–32% of SCLC patients.[31,34,38] Some studies have focused on antibodies against the SOX2 protein, which is highly similar both biochemically and functionally, showing comparable results. Interestingly, no patient with ataxia was reported in a prospective study of SOX2 antibodies, despite SOX being present in the human cerebellum.[39] For both SOX1 and SOX2 antibodies, no relation to any clinical or demographic characteristic has been found.[31,39]

SOX1 antibodies in LEMS

Upon first description of AGNA as a marker for paraneoplastic syndromes, the frequency of these antibodies was higher in LEMS, whereas no relation was found with other specific PNS subtypes.[33] AGNA was present in 43% of SCLC-LEMS patients compared to 12% of SCLC patients in general and not in NT-LEMS patients.[33] After identification of the antigen as SOX1 and refinement of specific antibody screening, two studies showed SOX1 antibodies to be present in 64–67% of patients with both SCLC and LEMS, compared to 0–5% positive NT-LEMS patients.[31,34] The frequency of SOX antibodies in both SCLC alone and SCLC with Hu antibodies was significantly lower, at 22–36% and 32–40%, respectively. Antibodies to HuD were detected in 30% of SCLC-LEMS patients and were only present in patients also positive for SOX antibodies (Fig. 1).[31] Development of an ELISA assay made testing for SOX antibodies amenable to high-throughput screening and available as a marker for

early tumor detection in newly diagnosed LEMS and other high-risk patients. Using this assay, SOX1 antibodies had a sensitivity of 67% and a specificity of 95% to discriminate between LEMS with associated SCLC and NT-LEMS.[31]

SOX antibodies have also been described in other disease entities, including neuropathy both of paraneoplastic and unknown origin without tumor on follow-up.[40] AGNA immunoreactivity has also been reported in two SCLC patients with limbic encephalitis associated with voltage-gated potassium channel (VGKC) antibodies.[41]

Effect of SOX1 and SOX2 antibodies on tumor survival was also studied in two separate studies, both for patients with SCLC-LEMS and SCLC alone. No survival effect of these onconeural antibodies was reported for either group (Fig. 2).[31,39] As for SOX antibodies in SCLC, no patient characteristics were related to the presence of SOX1 antibodies in SCLC-LEMS.[31] The lack of a survival effect or clinical difference between SOX-positive and -negative patients is not surprising considering SOX antibodies are directed against intracellular nuclear proteins. Since these intracellular proteins are not accessible to serum antibodies, a direct pathogenic role of SOX antibodies is unlikely.

SOX antibodies as marker for SCLC

SOX antibodies have also been investigated as immunobiomarker for early lung cancer detection. Antibodies against at least one marker in a panel of 6 SCLC-associated antigens were detected in 55% of SCLC patients, with a specificity of 90% as compared with controls matched for age, sex, and smoking history. Among the individual antigens studied, SOX2 antibodies were most frequent with a sensitivity and specificity of 35% and 97%, respectively.[42] Follow-up studies were conducted to validate a panel of six tumor-associated antigens to detect both small cell and non-SCLC.[43,44] This autoantibody panel showed a sensitivity of 36–39% and specificity of 89–91% for lung cancer as compared with matched controls in separate cohorts, which was confirmed in a second study using cohorts with specific tumor types. Low-sensitivity limits use of autoantibodies in screening for lung cancer; however, further refinement of specific immunobiomarkers tested in these panels could improve diagnostic yield in future studies.

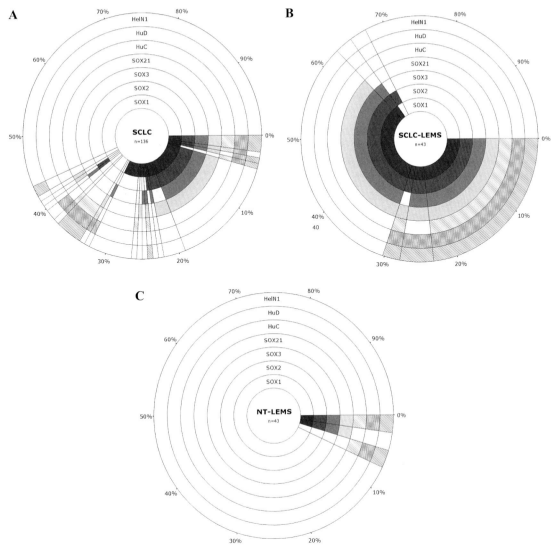

Figure 1. SOX and Hu-antibody responses in (A) SCLC patients without paraneoplastic syndrome; (B) SCLC-LEMS patients; and (C) nontumor LEMS patients. Reprinted with permission from Reference 31.

Tumor prediction in LEMS

Screening for SCLC after diagnosis of LEMS is very important as the tumor determines prognosis and treatment. Diagnosis of LEMS usually precedes tumor detection (94%), contributing to SCLC-LEMS patients being more likely to present with limited disease (65% in SCLC-LEMS vs. 39% in SCLC).[7] In SCLC-LEMS patients, the treatment will focus on tumor treatment to achieve improvement of both the tumor and neurological symptoms, whereas in moderate to severe NT-LEMS immunosuppressant drugs will be used as treatment.[2,45–47] Therefore,

the ability to predict which patients are at risk and which screening technique is most optimal has been investigated over the last years.

Clinical markers for tumor prediction

Several clinical markers have been described to discriminate between SCLC-LEMS and NT-LEMS, besides SOX antibodies as a serological marker. Although the frequency of specific clinical symptoms is comparable in both groups, LEMS has a more progressive course in patients with SCLC.[1,48,49] Subsequent symptoms occurred earlier in

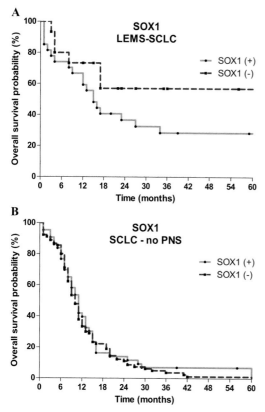

Figure 2. Survival of SOX1 (+) and SOX1 (−) small cell lung carcinoma (SCLC) patients with LEMS (A) or SCLC patients without PNS (B). Reprinted with permission from Reference 31.

SCLC-LEMS, especially distal weakness, bulbar, and autonomic symptoms.[48,49] Acute onset of muscle weakness is infrequent but has only been described in SCLC-LEMS.[1,48] Previously, O'Neill *et al.* described smoking history and age above 30 years as sensitive predictors of SCLC (96% and 100%, respectively), though specificity was moderate to very low (64% and 16%).[1] An increased erythrocyte sedimentation rate (ESR) showed similar prediction rates as did male gender.[1,14,45,48] The HLA haplotypes B8, DR3, and A1 are more frequently associated with NT-LEMS.[14] The combination of absence of HLA B8 and smoking history in LEMS patients had relatively good sensitivity (83%) and specificity (82%).[14] However, until recently, none of these factors seemed robust enough to guide screening methods in individual patients.

DELTA-P score

To increase the diagnostic yield, a dual cohort study was performed to aid in development of more reliable clinical screening tools.[8] First, a Dutch cohort of 107 LEMS patients was analyzed for variables associated with the presence of SCLC. Symptoms present in the first 3 months from onset of disease were used to develop a model to distinguish between SCLC-LEMS and NT-LEMS early in the course of the disease. This model was validated using a second cohort of 112 British LEMS patients. Clinical, genetic, and serological markers were investigated for all patients using univariate logistic regression to determine each variable's predictive value for SCLC. All factors significantly associated with SCLC were included in multivariate analysis to determine the most reliable and independent variables. Using the results of this multivariate model, the Dutch–English LEMS Tumor Association Prediction (DELTA-P) score was designed to predict the risk of subsequent SCLC detection in individual patients. Based on age at onset, smoking at onset, weight loss, Karnofsky performance status, bulbar symptoms, and male sexual impotence, all within 3 months of disease onset, it is our conclusion that this score indicates the presence of SCLC with very high accuracy (Fig. 3).[8] In both cohorts, the model was able to predict the likelihood of SCLC with higher than 94% reliability early in the course of their PNS. This prediction model, using only simple clinical markers, provides a tool to identify tumor risk and guide screening follow-up. A score of 0 or 1 virtually excludes an SCLC with a risk of 0% or 2.6%. A score of 3–6 should prompt intensive screening for SCLC, with a probability between 83.9% and 100% (Fig. 3).[8]

Screening for SCLC

Each patient should undergo primary tumor screening, even low-risk patients based on the DELTA-P score, as tumor detection has an important impact on treatment and prognosis. An associated SCLC is usually detected early after diagnosis of LEMS, 91% within 3 months, and 96% within a year.[7] Time intervals mentioned in the literature of more than 2 years between LEMS and tumor diagnosis were scarce and in patients with insufficient primary screening only. A follow-up study of a Dutch cohort of LEMS patients showed that CT-thorax is superior to chest X-ray.[7] CT-thorax detected 92% of lung tumors in SCLC-LEMS patients, 83% at first screening after LEMS diagnosis and an additional 9% at repeated screening, whereas X-rays only detected 43% of tumors.[7] FDG-PET scan has been shown to have an additional value for screening after diagnosis of LEMS and negative imaging studies.[7] This additional value has also been shown in screening of patients with other PNSs.[50–52] Bronchoscopy and mediastinoscopy are valuable for cytological or his-

tological diagnosis but were of no additional value if imaging techniques did not reveal any abnormalities.[7]

The DELTA-P score can be used to guide further screening methods in patients negative at first screening. We propose that patients at low risk (DELTA-P score 0–1) would have to undergo repeated screening only once 6 months after first screening (Fig. 4).[2] High-risk patients should have repeated screening after 3 months. If negative,

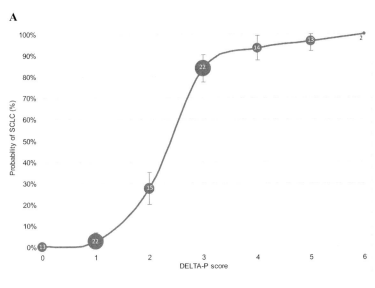

Figure 3. Predicted percentage of SLCL in patients with LEMS, based on the DELTA-P score. The DELTA-P score is calculated as a sum score according to the different categories listed. The DELTA-P score can range from 0 to 6. Point sizes proportionate to the number of patients with a specific score are also represented by the percentage inside the circle. Vertical bars indicate standard error of the mean SEM. Reprinted with permission from Reference 8.

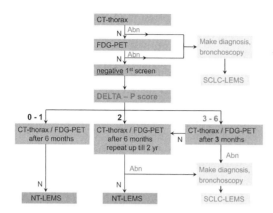

Figure 4. Flow chart for screening for SCLC. N, normal; Abn, abnormal. To screen for SCLC, the DELTA-P score (Fig. 3) can help to estimate the chance that an SCLC might be present. Reprinted with permission from Reference 2.

both intermediate- and high-risk patients should be screened every 6 months for 2 years after LEMS diagnosis.

Future directions

In conclusion, important advances have been made in increasing both our understanding of the immune mechanism and optimization of tumor screening in LEMS patients. SOX antibodies have been shown to be an important marker for SCLC-associated LEMS, though its significance in the immune response remains unclear. The DELTA-P score has provided for a simple clinical tool to indicate the presence of SCLC early in the course of LEMS. Future studies could further refine screening methods, which could prove of use for screening in other patients at high risk for lung cancer as well. Also, as for many autoimmune diseases, the precise mechanism responsible for triggering the immune response in both paraneoplastic and NT-LEMS remains unclear. The detailed insight in the pathophysiology and occurrence of both a paraneoplastic and nontumor form make LEMS an ideal candidate to study mechanisms of both general autoimmunity and tumor immunology.

Acknowledgments

This work is supported in part by the Prinses Beatrix Fonds (JJGMV). MJT is supported by a fellowship from the Dutch Cancer Society (KWF 2009–4451).

Conflicts of interest

The authors declare no conflicts of interest.

References

1. O'Neill, J.H., N.M. Murray & J. Newsom-Davis. 1988. The Lambert-Eaton myasthenic syndrome. A review of 50 cases. *Brain* **111**(Pt 3): 577–596.
2. Titulaer, M.J., B. Lang & J.J. Verschuuren. 2011. Lambert-Eaton myasthenic syndrome: from clinical characteristics to therapeutic strategies. *Lancet Neurol.* **10**: 1098–1107.
3. Motomura, M., I. Johnston, B. Lang, *et al.* 1995. An improved diagnostic assay for Lambert-Eaton myasthenic syndrome. *J. Neurol. Neurosurg. Psychiatry* **58**: 85–87.
4. Nakao, Y.K., M. Motomura, T. Fukudome, *et al.* 2002. Seronegative Lambert-Eaton myasthenic syndrome: study of 110 Japanese patients. *Neurology* **59**: 1773–1775.
5. Titulaer, M.J. & J.J. Verschuuren. 2008. Lambert-Eaton myasthenic syndrome: tumor versus nontumor forms. *Ann. N. Y. Acad. Sci.* **1132**: 129–134.
6. Wirtz, P.W., T.M. Smallegange, A.R. Wintzen, *et al.* 2002. Differences in clinical features between the Lambert-Eaton myasthenic syndrome with and without cancer: an analysis of 227 published cases. *Clin. Neurol. Neurosurg.* **104**: 359–363.
7. Titulaer, M.J., P.W. Wirtz, L.N. Willems, *et al.* 2008. Screening for small-cell lung cancer: a follow-up study of patients with Lambert-Eaton myasthenic syndrome. *J. Clin. Oncol.* **26**: 4276–4281.
8. Titulaer, M.J., P. Maddison, J.K. Sont, *et al.* 2011. Clinical Dutch-English Lambert-Eaton Myasthenic syndrome (LEMS) tumor association prediction score accurately predicts small-cell lung cancer in the LEMS. *J. Clin. Oncol.* **29**: 902–908.
9. Roberts, A., S. Perera, B. Lang, *et al.* 1985. Paraneoplastic myasthenic syndrome IgG inhibits 45Ca2+ flux in a human small cell carcinoma line. *Nature* **317**: 737–739.
10. Kaja, S., R.C. van de Ven, J.G. van Dijk, *et al.* 2007. Severely impaired neuromuscular synaptic transmission causes muscle weakness in the Cacna1a-mutant mouse rolling Nagoya. *Eur. J. Neurosci.* **25**: 2009–2020.
11. Lecky, B.R. 2006. Transient neonatal Lambert-Eaton syndrome. *J. Neurol. Neurosurg. Psychiatry* **77**: 1094.
12. Reuner, U., G. Kamin, G. Ramantani, *et al.* 2008. Transient neonatal Lambert-Eaton syndrome. *J. Neurol.* **255**: 1827–1828.
13. Wirtz, P.W., J. Bradshaw, A.R. Wintzen, *et al.* 2004. Associated autoimmune diseases in patients with the Lambert-Eaton myasthenic syndrome and their families. *J. Neurol.* **251**: 1255–1259.
14. Wirtz, P.W., N. Willcox, A.R. van der Slik, *et al.* 2005. HLA and smoking in prediction and prognosis of small cell lung cancer in autoimmune Lambert-Eaton myasthenic syndrome. *J. Neuroimmunol.* **159**: 230–237.
15. Price, P., C. Witt, R. Allcock, *et al.* 1999. The genetic basis for the association of the 8.1 ancestral haplotype (A1, B8, DR3) with multiple immunopathological diseases. *Immunol. Rev.* **167**: 257–274.
16. Compston, D.A., A. Vincent, J. Newsom-Davis, *et al.* 1980. Clinical, pathological, HLA antigen and immunological evidence for disease heterogeneity in myasthenia gravis. *Brain* **103**: 579–601.

17. Govindan, R., N. Page, D. Morgensztern, *et al.* 2006. Changing epidemiology of small-cell lung cancer in the United States over the last 30 years: analysis of the surveillance, epidemiologic, and end results database. *J. Clin. Oncol.* **24:** 4539–4544.

18. Tammemagi, C.M., C. Neslund-Dudas, M. Simoff, *et al.* 2004. Smoking and lung cancer survival: the role of comorbidity and treatment. *Chest* **125:** 27–37.

19. Delahunt, B., D.A. Abernethy, C.A. Johnson, *et al.* 2003. Prostate carcinoma and the Lambert-Eaton myasthenic syndrome. *J. Urol.* **169:** 278–279.

20. Wirtz, P.W., B. Lang, F. Graus, *et al.* 2005. P/Q-type calcium channel antibodies, Lambert-Eaton myasthenic syndrome and survival in small cell lung cancer. *J. Neuroimmunol.* **164:** 161–165.

21. Maddison, P., J. Newsom-Davis, K.R. Mills, *et al.* 1999. Favourable prognosis in Lambert-Eaton myasthenic syndrome and small-cell lung carcinoma. *Lancet* **353:** 117–118.

22. Maddison, P. & B. Lang. 2008. Paraneoplastic neurological autoimmunity and survival in small-cell lung cancer. *J. Neuroimmunol.* **201–202:** 159–162.

23. Graus, F., A. Saiz & J. Dalmau. 2010. Antibodies and neuronal autoimmune disorders of the CNS. *J. Neurol.* **257:** 509–517.

24. Deangelis, L.M. & J.B. Posner. 2008. *Neurologic Complications of Cancer.* Oxford University Press. Oxford.

25. Darnell, R.B. 1996. Onconeural antigens and the paraneoplastic neurologic disorders: at the intersection of cancer, immunity, and the brain. *Proc. Natl. Acad. Sci. USA* **93:** 4529–4536.

26. Campbell, A.M., B.G. Campling, K.M. Algazy, *et al.* 2002. Clinical and molecular features of small cell lung cancer. *Cancer Biol. Ther.* **1:** 105–112.

27. Darnell, R.B. & J.B. Posner. 2003. Paraneoplastic syndromes involving the nervous system. *N. Engl. J. Med.* **349:** 1543–1554.

28. Monstad, S.E., L. Drivsholm, A. Storstein, *et al.* 2004. Hu and voltage-gated calcium channel (VGCC) antibodies related to the prognosis of small-cell lung cancer. *J. Clin. Oncol.* **22:** 795–800.

29. Payne, M., P. Bradbury, B. Lang, *et al.* 2010. Prospective study into the incidence of Lambert Eaton myasthenic syndrome in small cell lung cancer. *J. Thorac. Oncol.* **5:** 34–38.

30. Graus, F., J. Dalmou, R. Rene, *et al.* 1997. Anti-Hu antibodies in patients with small-cell lung cancer: association with complete response to therapy and improved survival. *J. Clin. Oncol.* **15:** 2866–2872.

31. Titulaer, M.J., R. Klooster, M. Potman, *et al.* 2009. SOX antibodies in small-cell lung cancer and Lambert-Eaton myasthenic syndrome: frequency and relation with survival. *J. Clin. Oncol.* **27:** 4260–4267.

32. Gure, A.O., E. Stockert, M.J. Scanlan, *et al.* 2000. Serological identification of embryonic neural proteins as highly immunogenic tumor antigens in small cell lung cancer. *Proc. Natl. Acad. Sci. USA* **97:** 4198–4203.

33. Graus, F., A. Vincent, P. Pozo-Rosich, *et al.* 2005. Anti-glial nuclear antibody: marker of lung cancer-related paraneoplastic neurological syndromes. *J. Neuroimmunol.* **165:** 166–171.

34. Sabater, L., M. Titulaer, A. Saiz, *et al.* 2008. SOX1 antibodies are markers of paraneoplastic Lambert-Eaton myasthenic syndrome. *Neurology* **70:** 924–928.

35. Alcock, J., J. Lowe, T. England, *et al.* 2009. Expression of Sox1, Sox2 and Sox9 is maintained in adult human cerebellar cortex. *Neurosci. Lett.* **450:** 114–116.

36. Wegner, M. 2011. SOX after SOX: SOXession regulates neurogenesis. *Genes Dev.* **25:** 2423–2428.

37. Sholl, L.M., K.B. Long & J.L. Hornick. 2010. Sox2 expression in pulmonary non-small cell and neuroendocrine carcinomas. *Appl. Immunohistochem. Mol. Morphol.* **18:** 55–61.

38. Vural, B., L.C. Chen, P. Saip, *et al.* 2005. Frequency of SOX Group B (SOX1, 2, 3) and ZIC2 antibodies in Turkish patients with small cell lung carcinoma and their correlation with clinical parameters. *Cancer* **103:** 2575–2583.

39. Maddison, P., A. Thorpe, P. Silcocks, *et al.* 2010. Autoimmunity to SOX2, clinical phenotype and survival in patients with small-cell lung cancer. *Lung Cancer* **70:** 335–339.

40. Tschernatsch, M., P. Singh, O. Gross, *et al.* 2010. Anti-SOX1 antibodies in patients with paraneoplastic and non-paraneoplastic neuropathy. *J. Neuroimmunol.* **226:** 177–180.

41. Zuliani, L., A. Saiz, B. Tavolato, *et al.* 2007. Paraneoplastic limbic encephalitis associated with potassium channel antibodies: value of anti-glial nuclear antibodies in identifying the tumour. *J. Neurol. Neurosurg. Psychiatry* **78:** 204–205.

42. Chapman, C.J., A.J. Thorpe, A. Murray, *et al.* 2011. Immunobiomarkers in small cell lung cancer: potential early cancer signals. *Clin. Cancer Res.* **17:** 1474–1480.

43. Boyle, P., C.J. Chapman, S. Holdenrieder, *et al.* 2011. Clinical validation of an autoantibody test for lung cancer. *Ann. Oncol.* **22:** 383–389.

44. Lam, S., P. Boyle, G.F. Healey, *et al.* 2011. EarlyCDT-Lung: an immunobiomarker test as an aid to early detection of lung cancer. *Cancer Prev. Res. (Phila)* **4:** 1126–1134.

45. Sanders, D.B. 2003. Lambert-eaton myasthenic syndrome: diagnosis and treatment. *Ann. N.Y. Acad. Sci. USA* **998:** 500–508.

46. Chalk, C.H., N.M. Murray, J. Newsom-Davis, *et al.* 1990. Response of the Lambert-Eaton myasthenic syndrome to treatment of associated small-cell lung carcinoma. *Neurology* **40:** 1552–1556.

47. Maddison, P., B. Lang, K. Mills, *et al.* 2001. Long term outcome in Lambert-Eaton myasthenic syndrome without lung cancer. *J. Neurol. Neurosurg. Psychiatry* **70:** 212–217.

48. Wirtz, P.W., A.R. Wintzen & J.J. Verschuuren. 2005. Lambert-Eaton myasthenic syndrome has a more progressive course in patients with lung cancer. *Muscle Nerve* **32:** 226–229.

49. Titulaer, M.J., P.W. Wirtz, J.B. Kuks, *et al.* 2008. The Lambert-Eaton myasthenic syndrome 1988–2008: a clinical picture in 97 patients. *J. Neuroimmunol.* **201–202:** 153–158.

50. Linke, R., M. Schroeder, T. Helmberger, *et al.* 2004. Antibody-positive paraneoplastic neurologic syndromes: value of CT and PET for tumor diagnosis. *Neurology* **63:** 282–286.

51. Younes-Mhenni, S., M.F. Janier, L. Cinotti, *et al.* 2004. FDG-PET improves tumour detection in patients with paraneoplastic neurological syndromes. *Brain* **127:** 2331–2338.

52. Titulaer, M.J., R. Soffietti, J. Dalmau, *et al.* 2011. Screening for tumours in paraneoplastic syndromes: report of an EFNS task force. *Eur. J. Neurol.* **18:** 19-e3.

Ann. N.Y. Acad. Sci. ISSN 0077-8923

ANNALS OF THE NEW YORK ACADEMY OF SCIENCES

Issue: *Myasthenia Gravis and Related Disorders*

Treatment in Lambert–Eaton myasthenic syndrome

Paul Maddison

Department of Clinical Neurology, Queen's Medical Center, Nottingham, United Kingdom

Address for correspondence: Dr. Paul Maddison, Department of Clinical Neurology, Queen's Medical Center, Nottingham, NG7 2UH, United Kingdom. paul.maddison@nhs.net

Besides antitumor therapy for patients with the paraneoplastic form of Lambert–Eaton myasthenic syndrome (LEMS), the mainstay of symptomatic treatment in LEMS is 3,4-diaminopyridine (3,4-DAP). Data from four randomized, placebo-controlled trials have revealed that muscle strength scores increased significantly with 3,4-DAP. A limited meta-analysis performed on two trials using the Quantitative Myasthenia Gravis score indicated that the clinical benefits seen were modest. Meta-analysis of the mean change in compound muscle action potential amplitude following 3,4-DAP treatment revealed a significant improvement compared to placebo. However, most patients with noncancer LEMS require long-term immunosuppression, usually with prednisolone and azathioprine. A single crossover study has previously shown significant short-term benefit in limb strength following intravenous immunoglobulin, and there are isolated case reports of medium term benefit from rituximab. Overall, a combination of symptomatic treatment with 3,4-DAP and immunosuppression, with or without antitumor therapy, is often successful for most LEMS patients, with other more aggressive regimens rarely needed.

Keywords: treatment; Lambert–Eaton myasthenic syndrome; 3,4-diaminopyridine; steroids; meta-analysis

Introduction

Lambert–Eaton myasthenic syndrome (LEMS) is an autoimmune, presynaptic disorder of neuromuscular transmission characterized by proximal limb weakness, autonomic disturbance, depressed tendon reflexes, and posttetanic potentiation.[1,2] Approximately 50% of patients with LEMS have an underlying small-cell lung cancer (SCLC).[3,4] LEMS is an autoimmune disease mediated by antibodies to P/Q-type voltage-gated calcium channels (VGCC) at the motor nerve terminal.[5–7] Treatment is based around anticancer therapy for those patients with associated tumors, often given in conjunction with (and solely for patients with noncancer LEMS) both symptomatic treatment and immunosuppression.

Symptomatic treatment

Given that LEMS is a presynaptic disorder characterized by impaired quantal release of acetylcholine, symptomatic treatment has used drugs that increase neurotransmitter release at the neuromuscular junction.

Guanidine

Guanidine was first recommended for use in LEMS by Lambert[8] but has not been used in large randomized controlled trials because of serious side effects of marrow suppression[9] and renal failure.[10] However, low dose guanidine (less than 1,000 mg/day) has been used in conjunction with pyridostigmine in one small open-labeled study that resulted in improved muscle strength and neurophysiological measurements in all nine LEMS patients studied.[11] One third of these study patients had to discontinue guanidine due to persistent gastrointestinal side effects.

4-Aminopyridine

The quaternary ammonium compound, 4-aminopyridine (4-AP), was found to increase the release of acetylcholine at the neuromuscular junction[12] and was therefore subsequently used for the symptomatic treatment of two patients with LEMS.[13,14] A larger open study of the use of oral 4-AP in four patients with LEMS resulted in clinical and electrophysiological improvement, but one participant suffered a single generalized seizure while taking a

doi: 10.1111/j.1749-6632.2012.06769.x

dose of 120 mg 4-AP per day.[15] The possibility of significant central nervous system side effects such as seizures has therefore limited the use of 4-AP, a drug known to cross the blood–brain barrier and result in epileptogenic effects in animals.[16]

3,4-Diaminopyridine

The related aminopyridine 3,4-diaminopyridine (3,4-DAP) has become the mainstay of symptomatic treatment for LEMS in Europe, with the phosphate salt preparation amifampridine recently receiving a European license for treatment in LEMS.[17] 3,4-DAP has been shown in animals to be more potent in improving neuromuscular transmission[18] and less convulsant[19] than 4-AP. In addition, it has the advantage over 4-AP of crossing the blood–brain barrier less readily,[20] resulting in fewer central nervous system side effects. Although initially thought to act solely by blocking voltage-gated potassium channels, thus prolonging the action potential at the motor nerve terminal and lengthening the VGCC opening time, recent data have suggested that 3,4-DAP may also potentiate neuromuscular transmission by direct effects on the VGCC beta subunit.[21]

The first use of 3,4-DAP was in three patients with LEMS without lung cancer who all improved clinically and electrophysiologically from intravenous and then oral preparations of 3,4-DAP.[22] Follow-up data collected after a mean treatment duration of five years demonstrated prolonged clinical benefit with few side effects at daily doses less than 60 mg of 3,4-DAP.[23]

Since these initial reports, there have been a number of additional trials of 3,4-DAP in LEMS. To date, there have been four randomized placebo-controlled trials of 3,4-DAP in a total of 54 patients with LEMS.[24–27] No trial involved healthy or disease control groups.

The first 3,4-DAP trial to be published was a crossover trial of 12 participants comparing the effect of maximum dose oral 3,4-DAP (100 mg/day) for six days with placebo, using a muscle strength score and electrophysiological testing at three and six days.[24] The authors found a significant improvement in isometric muscle strength and a parallel increase in resting compound muscle action potential (CMAP) amplitudes following 3,4-DAP treatment in all participants compared with placebo.

A second trial with a parallel group design compared oral 3,4-DAP (60 mg/day) with placebo (oral lactose capsules) in 26 participants (12 received 3,4-DAP, 14 placebo).[27] A Quantitative Myasthenia Gravis (QMG)[28] muscle strength score and electrophysiological measurements were taken on days five and six. The authors demonstrated a significant improvement in both the QMG muscle strength score and summated median CMAP amplitude after six days in patients taking 3,4-DAP compared to placebo.

The third trial reported was a placebo-controlled, double-dummy, double-blind, randomized crossover study of nine patients with LEMS in which the study group compared 10 mg of intravenous 3,4-DAP with placebo infusion, i.v. pyridostigmine (varying doses), and a combination of 3,4-DAP and pyridostigmine.[25] Isometric muscle strength of hip flexion, measured by dynamometry, and resting CMAP amplitude from the hypothenar eminence were recorded every 20 min between 10 and 170 min postinfusion. The authors found that both CMAP amplitude and isometric muscle strength increased significantly during treatment with 3,4-DAP compared with placebo. The addition of pyridostigmine to 3,4-DAP did not confer any additional benefit, and treatment with pyridostigmine alone did not improve CMAP amplitude and isometric muscle strength compared with placebo.

The fourth, and latest, trial published was a randomized, double blind, placebo-controlled, crossover study oral 3,4-DAP in seven patients with LEMS.[26] The treatment protocol varied, with the first group of three cases treated with an initial daily dose of 15 mg increasing to 80 mg per day by the end of the eight-day period. A second group was treated with 30 mg per day increasing to 75 mg/day over a three-day study period due to time constraints. Endpoints included a subjective symptoms score, LEMS classification, Medical Research Council (MRC) summated muscle strength score, QMG score, abductor digiti quinti (ADQ) CMAP amplitude, and repetitive nerve stimulation. All four clinical scores improved significantly with 3,4-DAP compared with placebo, as did resting ADQ CMAP amplitudes after 6–16 days.

Extended follow-up of 12–21 months by McEvoy et al.[24] showed sustained benefit in favor of 3,4-DAP. Almost all (22 of 25) participants studied by Sanders et al.[27] gained sustained benefit from

A

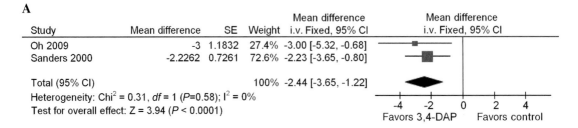

B

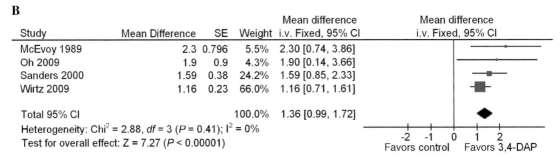

Figure 1. (A) Meta-analysis of the change in QMG score with 3,4-diaminopyridine (3,4-DAP) treatment using generic inverse variance method. (B) Meta-analysis of the change in mean compound muscle action potential amplitude (mV) with 3,4-diaminopyridine (3,4-DAP) treatment using generic inverse variance method.

3,4-DAP treatment over a six-month follow-up period. Oh *et al.*[26] described patients' choice for long-term treatment at the cessation of the trial, and gave a subjective or objective account of their progress.

All four randomized trials of 3,4-DAP reported a significant improvement in either muscle strength score, or myometric limb measurement following treatment. However, a meta-analysis of these results from all four studies was not possible because of marked differences between these trials regarding primary outcome measures.[29] Meta-analysis on QMG scores based on the data provided in the papers by Sanders *et al.*[27] and Oh *et al.*[26] showed that QMG score improved with 3,4-DAP treatment compared to baseline QMG values, with a mean overall improvement of 2.44 points, (95% CI: 1.22–3.6 points) (generic inverse variance [GIV] analysis, Fig. 1A).

All trials recorded changes in the amplitude of resting CMAPs after active treatment or placebo. Meta-analysis of the CMAP secondary endpoint showed a significant overall benefit in CMAP amplitude after treatment with 3,4-DAP.[29] The overall mean improvement on GIV analysis was 1.36 mV (95% CI: 0.99–1.72), in favor of the treatment (Fig. 1B). In the analyses of the effects of 3,4-DAP treatment in three trials, the numbers of patients with an

associated SCLC ($n = 15$) was too small to enable statistically meaningful subgroup analysis.

Major adverse events from 3,4-DAP are seldom encountered.[24–27,30] Mild, common side effects include brief perioral tingling and acral paresthesias, fatigue, insomnia, abdominal pain, anxiety, blurred vision, diarrhea, dizziness, palpitiations, and epigastric discomfort. One patient suffered from a seizure after 10 months of 3,4-DAP treatment.[24] This occurred soon after her daily dose of 3,4-DAP was increased from 90 mg to 100 mg, and her pyridostigmine dose doubled to 240 mg a day, and never recurred when the daily dose of 3,4-DAP was reduced to 40 mg. It has thus been recommended by some authors that the dose of 3,4-DAP in LEMS patients is limited to 80 mg per day.[27] Monitoring of routine blood tests, electrocardiography, and electroencephalography does not typically reveal any abnormalities during 3,4-DAP treatment.[24,27]

Pyridostigmine

Although in practice some patients with LEMS may report an additional clinical benefit when adding pyridostigmine to 3,4-DAP,[24,31] data from a small, clinical study of intravenous preparations have failed to suggest an objective additional benefit when pyridostigmine is added to 3,4-DAP.[25]

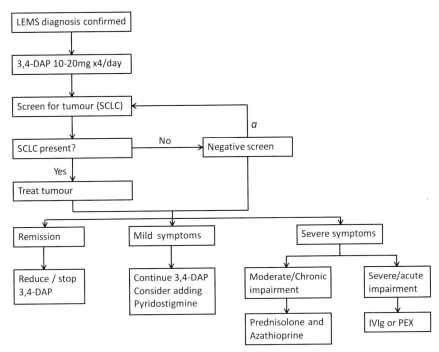

Figure 2. Adapted treatment schedule for LEMS.[44] SCLC, small-cell lung cancer; IVIg, intravenous immunoglobulin; PEX, plasma exchange.[a]Number of repeat screenings required as per previously published guidelines.[45]

Immunosuppression

Acute treatment

Plasma exchange, usually delivered as a five-day course, removing 3–4 L on each day, typically improves LEMS symptoms and objective CMAP amplitude outcome measures promptly, in both cancer and noncancer LEMS. The peak beneficial effect is usually demonstrated after about two weeks, largely subsiding after six weeks.[32]

Short-term beneficial effects were also observed in a single randomized placebo-controlled crossover study of intravenous immunoglobulin (IVIg) (total 2 g/kg body weight over two days) in nine noncancer LEMS patients, with significant improvement in the primary outcome of limb strength (measured by myometry), peaking at two to four weeks, and declining by eight weeks. All patients had stable disease, and were previously treated with oral immunosuppression.[33] One patient in this study developed acute meningism after IVIg, which did not recur on treatment retrial. There are no objective data to support the long term, intermittent use of IVIg in LEMS.

Long-term treatment

In patients whose LEMS symptoms are not adequately controlled on symptomatic treatment, long-term oral immunosuppression with prednisolone and azathioprine is usually considered, with treatment regimens based on previous trial data in myasthenia gravis (prednisolone increasing initially from 10 mg on alternate days, by 10 mg every other day, up to 1.5 mg/kg (or 100 mg whichever dose was smaller) on alternate days; azathioprine 50 mg per day, increasing by 25 mg per day to a total dose of 2.5 mg/kg per day) showing beneficial effects from combined therapy.[34] Retrospective, observational follow-up data on 47 noncancer LEMS patients in one center demonstrated that combination therapy of prednisolone and azathioprine was required in almost all patients (approximately 90%), with 43% achieving sustained clinical remission within the first three years of treatment.[35] However, significant doses of prednisolone (mean 30 mg (median 25 mg) on alternate days, often combined with azathioprine) were still required after three years' follow-up, with only 14% achieving clinical and pharmacological remission. In this series, muscle strength scores were improved in 88% of patients after a median duration of immunosuppressive treatment of six years; anti-VGCC antibody titres fell in half the patients, and mean resting CMAP amplitudes improved to normal values after two years of treatment.[35] These findings are in concordance with data from other centers where observational studies on 73 LEMS patients (31 with lung cancer) have previously demonstrated that high-dose prednisolone often only achieved mild to moderate improvement in symptoms, which was not sustained when the dose was reduced.[31,36] Oral immunosuppression seems to be effective for patients with cancer-LEMS, but successful antineoplastic therapy is of greater importance.[37]

To date, two patients with severe symptoms of LEMS, resistant to multiple oral immunosuppressant agents, have been treated with Rituximab with marked clinical benefit at one year, but short of remission.[38] No significant side effects were observed. There are no long-term data on the effects of Rituximab in LEMS, given either as an initial series of injections, or repeated courses.

Antitumor therapy

As approximately half of all LEMS patients have an underlying tumor (usually SCLC), and the symptoms of LEMS almost invariably occur before the discovery of the malignancy, screening for SCLC is of paramount importance at the point of LEMS diagnosis (Fig. 2). Clinical prediction scores for the development of SCLC, and SCLC screening protocols have now been validated and published.[39,40] Specific antitumor therapy often improves LEMS symptoms, perhaps by reducing the antigenic stimulus from the tumor, as it is thought that tumor surface VGCCs provoke the anti-VGCC antibody response.[41] In one series, 7 of 11 SCLC–LEMS patients who survived antitumor therapy (chemotherapy, and in some, radiotherapy) by two months or longer, subsequently showed progressive improvement in their LEMS symptoms.[37] All these patients were taking symptomatic treatment (3,4-DAP), and although half required maintenance immunosuppression with prednisolone, the marked initial and subsequently sustained clinical and electromyographical improvement observed paralleled the use of antitumor therapy. Long-term clinical and pharmacological remission has been reported in patients following successful SCLC resection.[37]

Discussion

Symptomatic 3,4-DAP treatment has been shown to be well tolerated and effective for patients with LEMS with or without an associated cancer. In a limited meta-analysis of the effects of 3,4-DAP in LEMS,[29] the apparent improvement in QMG score in two trials must be placed in the context of the reliability of the QMG score as a primary efficacy measurement in clinical trials as outlined by Barohn et al.[28] The QMG score in these validation studies was principally designed for patients with myasthenia gravis, and the score changes judged to be a meaningful clinical improvement were not calculated in patients with LEMS. The other two primary endpoint clinical scores have never been validated in further studies. The use of a uniform primary outcome clinical measure, ideally adapted and validated for LEMS, in future trials would enable a more definitive treatment effect to be established with meta-analysis.

Owing to the rare occurrence of seizures in LEMS patients treated with 3,4-DAP, usually at a daily dose of 100 mg, it has been recommended that the daily oral dose of 3,4-DAP should not exceed 80 mg.[27] This would seem to be a reasonable recommendation given that most patients in the four reported randomized trials received doses of oral (or intravenous equivalent) 3,4-DAP lower than 100 mg per day, with clinical and electrophysiological improvement. No cardiac abnormalities were encountered in the trials at these doses of 3,4-DAP, as would be expected, considering the only case reported in detail of cardiac side effects (supraventricular tachyarrhythmia) in a patient taking 3,4-DAP for LEMS occurred in a patient given an erroneously high daily dose of 360 mg.[42] Alternative symptomatic therapies are being developed for LEMS, including the novel calcium channel agonist GV-359–58, a derivative of roscovitine.[43] However, the data on physiological effects have only been reported on mouse passive transfer experiments, and the clinical benefits and potential side effects in humans is, as yet, unknown.

Specific antitumor therapy often improves LEMS symptoms significantly, and thus vigilance for the development of SCLC in particular would remain paramount. There are validated clinical SCLC prediction scores, and screening paradigms now available.[39,40] Although acute treatment with IVIg or plasma exchange is only seldom required for severe

LEMS symptoms, achievement and maintenance of clinical remission requires substantial doses of oral immunosuppression, and thus evaluation of alternative treatments such as rituximab may be warranted.

Acknowledgments

Figure 1A and B is based in part on a Cochrane Review published in the Cochrane Library 2011, Issue 2 (see www.thecochranelibrary.com for information). Cochrane Reviews are regularly updated as new evidence emerges and in response to feedback, and the Cochrane Library should be consulted for the most recent version of the review.

Conflicts of interest

P.M. received a single honorarium for consultancy work from BioMarin.

References

1. Lambert, E.H., L.M. Eaton & E.D. Rooke. 1956. Defect of neuromuscular conduction associated with malignant neoplasms. *Am. J. Physiol.* **187:** 612–613.
2. Lambert, E.H. & D. Elmqvist. 1971. Quantal components of end-plate potentials in the myasthenic syndrome. *Ann. N.Y. Acad. Sci.* **183:** 183–199.
3. O'Neill, J.H., N.M.F. Murray & J. Newsom-Davis. 1988. The Lambert-Eaton myasthenic syndrome: a review of 50 cases. *Brain* **111:** 577–596.
4. Wirtz, P.W., J.G. van Dijk, P.A. van Doorn, *et al.* 2004. The epidemiology of the Lambert-Eaton myasthenic syndrome in the Netherlands. *Neurology* **63:** 397–398.
5. Lang, B., J. Newsom-Davis, D. Wray, *et al.* 1981. Autoimmune aetiology for myasthenic (Eaton-Lambert) syndrome. *Lancet* **2:** 224–226.
6. Lennon, V.A., T.J. Kryzer, G.E. Griesmann, *et al.* 1995. Calcium-channel antibodies in the Lambert-Eaton syndrome and other paraneoplastic syndromes. *N. Engl. J. Med.* **332:** 1467–1474.
7. Motomura, M., I. Johnston, B. Lang, *et al.* 1995. An improved diagnostic assay for Lambert-Eaton myasthenic syndrome. *J. Neurol. Neurosurg. Psychiatry* **58:** 85–87.
8. Lambert, E.H. 1966. Defects of neuromuscular transmission in syndromes other than myasthenia gravis. *Ann. N.Y. Acad. Sci.* **135:** 367–384.
9. Oh, S.J. & K.W. Kim. 1973. Guanidine hydrochloride in the Eaton-Lambert syndrome. Electrophysiologic improvement. *Neurology* **23:** 1084–1090.
10. Blumhardt, L.D., A.M. Joekes, J. Marshall & P.E. Philalithis. 1977. Guanidine treatment and impaired renal function in the Eaton-Lambert syndrome. *BMJ* **1:** 946–947.
11. Oh, S.J., D.S. Kim, T.C. Head & G.C. Claussen. 1997. Low-dose guanidine and pyridostigmine: relatively safe and effective long-term symptomatic therapy in Lambert-Eaton myasthenic syndrome. *Muscle Nerve* **20:** 1146–1152.
12. Lundh, H. 1978. Effects of 4-aminopyridine on neuromuscular transmission. *Brain Res.* **153:** 307–318.
13. Lundh, H., O. Nilsson & I. Rosén. 1977. 4-Aminopyridine—a new drug tested in the treatment of Eaton-Lambert syndrome. *J. Neurol. Neurosurg. Psychiatry* **40:** 1109–1112.
14. Agoston, S., T. van Weerden, P. Westra & A. Broekert. 1978. Effects of 4-aminopyridine in Eaton Lambert Syndrome. *Br. J. Anaesth.* **50:** 383–385.
15. Murray, N.M.F. & J. Newsom-Davis. 1981. Treatment with oral 4-aminopyridine in disorders of neuromuscular transmission. *Neurology* **31:** 265–271.
16. Lemeignan, M. 1971. Pharmacological approach to the study of convulsive action mechanism of amino-4 pyridine [Abord pharmacologique de l'étude du mécanisme de l'action convulsivante de l'amino-4 pyridine]. *Therapie* **26:** 927–940.
17. BioMarin Europe Ltd. Summary of Product Characteristics. Firdapse® (amifampridine). Date of Preparation of Text January 2010.
18. Molgó, J., H. Lundh & S. Thesleff. 1980. Potency of 3,4-diaminopyridine and 4-aminopyridine on mammalian neuromuscular transmission and the effect of pH changes. *Eur. J. Pharmacol.* **61:** 25–34.
19. Lechat, P., G. Deysson, M. Lemeignan & M. Adolphe. 1968. Comparison of acute toxicity of some aminopyridines in vivo (mice) and in vitro (tissue culture) [Toxicité aigue composareé de quelques aminopyridines in vivo (souris) et in vitro (cultures cellulaires)]. *Ann. Pharm. Fr.* **26:** 345–349.
20. Lemeignan, M., H. Millart, N. Letteron, *et al.* 1982. The ability of 4-aminopyridine and 3,4-diaminopyridine to cross the blood-brain barrier can account for their difference in toxicity. In *Aminopyridines and Similarly Acting Drugs: Effects on Nerves, Muscles and Synapses. Advances in the Biosciences.* Vol. 35. P. Lechat, S. Thesleff & W.C. Bowman, Eds.: 222–229. Pergamon Press. Oxford.
21. Wu, Z.Z., D.P. Li, S.R. Chen & H.L. Pan. 2009. Aminopyridines potentiate synaptic and neuromuscular transmission by targeting the voltage-activated calcium channel beta subunit. *J. Biol. Chem.* **284:** 36453–36461.
22. Lundh, H., O. Nilsson & I. Rosén. 1983. Novel drug of choice in Eaton-Lambert syndrome. *J. Neurol. Neurosurg. Psychiatry* **46:** 684–685.
23. Lundh, H., O. Nilsson, I. Rosén & S. Johansson. 1993. Practical aspects of 3,4-diaminopyridine treatment of the Lambert-Eaton myasthenic syndrome. *Acta. Neurol. Scand.* **88:** 136–140.
24. McEvoy, K.M., A.J. Windebank, J.R. Daube & P.A. Low. 1989. 3,4-Diaminopyridine in the treatment of Lambert-Eaton myasthenic syndrome. *N. Engl. J. Med.* **321:** 1567–1571.
25. Wirtz, P.W., J.J. Verschuuren, J.G. van Dijk, *et al.* 2009. Efficacy of 3,4-diaminopyridine and pyridostigmine in the treatment of Lambert-Eaton myasthenic syndrome: a randomized, double-blind, placebo-controlled, cross-over study. *Clin. Pharmacol. Ther.* **86:** 44–48.
26. Oh, S.J., G.G. Claussen, Y. Hatanaka & M.B. Morgan. 2009. 3,4-diaminopyridine is more effective than placebo in a randomized, double-blind, cross-over drug study in LEMS. *Muscle Nerve* **40:** 795–800.
27. Sanders, D.B., J.M. Massey, L.L. Sanders & L.J. Edwards. 2000. A randomized trial of 3,4-diaminopyridine in

Lambert-Eaton myasthenic syndrome. *Neurology* **54:** 603–607.

28. Barohn, R.J., D. McIntire, L. Herbelin, *et al.* 1998. Reliability testing of the quantitative myasthenia gravis score. *Ann. N.Y. Acad. Sci.* **841:** 769–772.

29. Keogh, M., S. Sedehizadeh & P. Maddison. 2011. Treatment for Lambert-Eaton myasthenic syndrome. *Cochrane Database Syst. Rev.* **2:** CD003279.

30. Wirtz, P.W., M.J. Titulaer, J.M.A. van Gerven & J.J. Verschuuren. 2010. 3,4-diaminopyridine for the treatment of Lambert-Eaton myasthenic syndrome. *Exp. Rev. Clin. Immunol.* **6:** 867–874.

31. Tim, R.W., J.M. Massey & D.B. Sanders. 2000. Lambert-Eaton myasthenic syndrome: electrodiagnostic findings and response to treatment. *Neurology* **54:** 2176–2178.

32. Newsom-Davis, J. & N.M.F. Murray. 1984. Plasma exchange and immunosuppressive drug treatment in Lambert-Eaton myasthenic syndrome. *Neurology* **34:** 480–485.

33. Bain, P.G., M. Motomura, J. Newsom-Davis, *et al.* 1996. Effects of intravenous immunoglobulin on muscle weakness and calcium-channel autoantibodies in the Lambert-Eaton myasthenic syndrome. *Neurology* **47:** 678–683.

34. Palace, J., J. Newsom-Davis & B. Lecky. 1998. A randomized double-blind trial of prednisolone alone or with azathioprine in myasthenia gravis. Myasthenia Gravis Study Group. *Neurology* **50:** 1778–1783.

35. Maddison, P., B. Lang, K. Mills & J. Newsom-Davis. 2001. Long term outcome in Lambert-Eaton myasthenic syndrome without lung cancer. *J. Neurol. Neurosurg. Psychiatry* **70:** 212–217.

36. Tim, R.W., J.M. Massey & D.B. Sanders. 1998. Lambert-Eaton myasthenic syndrome (LEMS). Clinical and electrodiagnostic features and response to therapy in 59 patients. *Ann. N.Y. Acad. Sci.* **841:** 823–826.

37. Chalk, C.H., N.M. Murray, J. Newsom-Davis, *et al.* 1990.

Response of the Lambert-Eaton myasthenic syndrome to treatment of associated small-cell lung carcinoma. *Neurology.* **40:** 1552–1556.

38. Maddison, P., J. McConville, M.E. Farrugia, *et al.* 2011. The use of rituximab in myasthenia gravis and Lambert-Eaton myasthenic syndrome. *J. Neurol. Neurosurg. Psychiatry* **82:** 671–673.

39. Titulaer, M.J., R. Soffietti, J. Dalmau, *et al.*European Federation of Neurological Societies. 2011. Screening for tumors in paraneoplastic syndromes: report of an EFNS task force. *Eur. J. Neurol.* **18:** 19-e3.

40. Titulaer, M.J., P. Maddison, J.K. Sont, *et al.* 2011. Clinical Dutch-English Lambert-Eaton Myasthenic syndrome (LEMS) tumor association prediction score accurately predicts small-cell lung cancer in the LEMS. *J. Clin. Oncol.* **29:** 902–908.

41. Roberts, A., S. Perera, B. Lang, *et al.* 1985. Paraneoplastic myasthenic syndrome IgG inhibits 45Ca2+ flux in a human small cell carcinoma line. *Nature* **317:** 737–739.

42. Boerma, C.E., J.H. Rommes, R.B. van Leeuwen & J. Bakker. 1995. Cardiac arrest following an iatrogenic 3,4-diaminopyridine intoxication in a patient with Lambert-Eaton myasthenic syndrome. *J. Toxicol. Clin. Toxicol.* **33:** 249–251.

43. Tarr, T.B., G. Valdomir, M. Liang, P. Wipf & S.D. Meriney. 2012. New calcium channel agonists as potential therapeutics in Lambert-Eaton myasthenic syndrome and other neuromuscular diseases. *Ann. N.Y. Acad. Sci.* **1275:** 85–91.

44. Newsom-Davis, J. 1998. A treatment algorithm for Lambert-Eaton myasthenic syndrome. *Ann. N.Y. Acad. Sci.* **841:** 817–822.

45. Titulaer, M.J., B Lang & J.J. Verschuuren. 2011. Lambert-Eaton myasthenic syndrome: from clinical characteristics to therapeutic strategies. *Lancet Neurol.* **10:** 1098–1107.

Ann. N.Y. Acad. Sci. ISSN 0077-8923

New calcium channel agonists as potential therapeutics in Lambert–Eaton myasthenic syndrome and other neuromuscular diseases

Tyler B. Tarr,[1] Guillermo Valdomir,[2] Mary Liang,[2] Peter Wipf,[2] and Stephen D. Meriney[1]

[1]Department of Neuroscience, [2]Department of Chemistry, University of Pittsburgh, Pittsburgh, Pennsylvania

Address for correspondence: Stephen D. Meriney, Department of Neuroscience, A210 Langley Hall, University of Pittsburgh, Pittsburgh, PA 15260. meriney@pitt.edu

Lambert–Eaton myasthenic syndrome (LEMS) causes neuromuscular weakness as a result of an autoimmune attack on the calcium channels that normally regulate chemical transmitter release at the neuromuscular junction. Currently there are limited treatment options for patients with this and other forms of neuromuscular weakness. A novel, first-in-class calcium channel agonist that is selective for the types of voltage-gated calcium channels that regulate transmitter release at neuromuscular synapses has recently been developed. This compound (GV-58) slows deactivation (closing) of the channel, resulting in a large increase in total calcium entry during motor nerve action potential activity. This new calcium channel agonist is currently being evaluated for the treatment of neuromuscular weakness. Potential applications include development as single therapeutics, or for combination treatments.

Keywords: calcium channel; transmitter release; Lambert–Eaton myasthenic syndrome; roscovitine

Lambert–Eaton myasthenic syndrome (LEMS) is an autoantibody-mediated disorder of the neuromuscular junction that is often associated with small cell lung cancer.[1–3] LEMS is characterized by a progressive muscle weakness that affects everyday activities and quality of life, with a prevalence of about 2–4 cases per million.[2,4] LEMS symptoms have been shown to be caused by a decrease in quantal content of transmitter release from the neuromuscular junction,[5] which is caused by an autoimmune-mediated removal of presynaptic calcium channels.[6,7] The presence of antibodies to other presynaptic proteins may occur and contribute to an existing presynaptic neuromuscular weakness.[8–10] Based on studies in LEMS-model mice, it is hypothesized that motoneurons attempt to compensate for this autoantibody-mediated attack by upregulating the expression of several types of calcium channels,[11] but overall, passive transfer of LEMS to mice results in decreased presynaptic calcium entry during an action potential.[12] There is no cure for LEMS, and few treatment options

are available. If cancer is present, antitumor therapy is the priority. In any case, this type of neuromuscular weakness can be treated using either immunosuppressants or symptomatic treatment approaches. Immunosuppressants have not been favored, as side effects may be severe and include leukopenia, liver dysfunction, nausea, and vomiting.[13] Symptomatic treatment strategies that increase transmitter release have emerged as the primary therapeutic approach and are currently recommended.[13,14] Commonly, a potassium channel blocker is used alone or, alternatively, in combination with an acetylcholinesterase inhibitor.[15–17] In clinical trials, 10–20 mg of the potassium channel blocker 3,4-diaminopyridine (DAP), which increases calcium entry by broadening the action potential depolarization, was given three times per day and led to serum levels of about 0.5–1 μM.[15,16] In these studies, DAP treatment was shown to be effective, leading to significant improvement in muscle strength and compound muscle action potential (CMAP) amplitude in LEMS patients.

doi: 10.1111/nyas.12001

However, although it is generally well tolerated, DAP can have side effects that include paresthesia, gastric symptoms, difficulty in sleeping, fatigue, and deterioration of muscle strength.[14,16] The latter two may be due to reported effects on axonal K^+ channels that limit firing frequencies,[18] and/or reduction in activity-dependent facilitation caused by DAP.[19] Thus, the current LEMS treatment approach indirectly increases calcium entry into the nerve terminal. In an attempt to develop alternative therapeutic options, a novel strategy would be to target directly the calcium channels that regulate transmitter release. Recently, calcium channel gating modifiers with promise for treatment of neuromuscular disorders have been developed based on the parent molecule *R*-roscovitine.[20,21]

R-roscovitine as a lead in the development of novel calcium channel agonists

R-Roscovitine is a trisubstituted purine that is best known as an inhibitor of cyclin-dependent kinases

(cdks). Cdks have been implicated in neuronal development,[22] synaptic transmission,[23] cytoskeletal control,[24,25] neurodegeneration,[26] and cell cycle control.[27] In terms of clinical use, some inhibitors of cdks are being tested for use as anticancer drugs and in the treatment of neurodegenerative diseases.[28] Roscovitine is a chiral compound, and both *R* and *S* configurations are effective cdk inhibitors. Interestingly, *R*-roscovitine has effects on targets independent of its effects on cdks, including a direct action on a subset of voltage-gated calcium channels.[29–31] *R*-Roscovitine binds selectively to the open configuration of P/Q- and N-type calcium channels, slowing their deactivation kinetics and increasing total calcium entry.[29,32,33] The effects of *R*-roscovitine have also previously been characterized on N-type Ca^{2+} channel currents in frog motoneurons[31] and tsA-201 cell lines expressing mammalian N-type or P/Q-type Ca^{2+} channels (Fig. 1).[34] Furthermore, at the single channel level, it is known that calcium channels normally gate with a short (predominant)

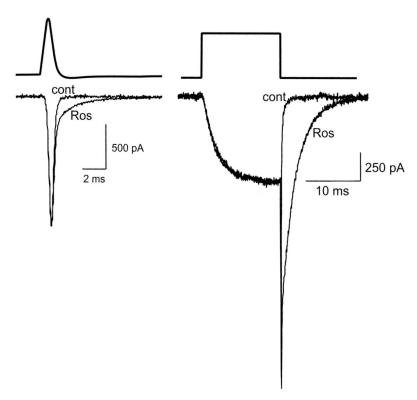

Figure 1. Effects of 100 μM *R*-roscovitine on P/Q-type currents recorded from tsA-201 cells. Current is evoked by an action potential–like waveform (left panel; from −100 mV to +25 mV at the peak), and a step depolarization (right panel; from −100 mV to +10 mV). In both panels, the top trace is the voltage waveform and the bottom trace is calcium current under control (cont) or *R*-roscovitine–treated (Ros) conditions.

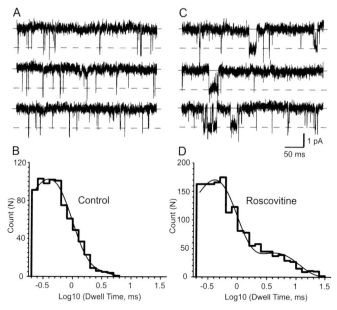

Figure 2. *R*-Roscovitine prolongs mean open time of N-type calcium channels expressed in tsA-201 cells and increases the probability of observing channels opening with long open time. (A) Sample control openings evoked by voltage steps from −120 to −30 mV. (B) Open time distribution for a representative control patch is best fit by the sum of two exponentials, with short openings predominant. (C) Representative sweeps from an (*R*)-roscovitine–exposed patch. Under these conditions, a combination of short and long openings is observed. (D) Open time distribution for a representative (*R*)-roscovitine–treated patch is best fit by the sum of two exponentials, but the longer component is prolonged (compared to control) and more evident than in control (untreated) patches. Adapted from DeStefino *et al.*[34]

or long (rare) mean open time. It has been shown that *R*-roscovitine significantly prolongs the mean open time of calcium channels gating with a long open time, and increases the probability of observing channels that gate with a long open time (Fig. 2).[34] These effects lead to increased calcium flux when channels are naturally activated by an action potential, which increases transmitter release at neuromuscular and CNS synapses.[29,31] The effect of *R*-roscovitine on calcium channels is the basis for recent work aimed at developing analogs of this drug as potential treatments for motor nerve terminal dysfunction. The goal has been to develop *R*-roscovitine analogs with reduced cdk activity and stronger, higher affinity calcium channel agonist effects that would be appropriate to treat neuromuscular weakness.

cently, Liang *et al.*[21] reported the synthesis and assay of more than 20 analogs of *R*-roscovitine. The most promising analog that emerged from these studies (GV-58; compound "13x" in Liang *et al.*[21]) was reported to have greater than 20-fold lower cdk activity and three- to fourfold higher affinity for calcium channels.[20,21] Additionally, it is approximately fourfold more potent as a calcium channel agonist than *R*-roscovitine. Significantly, GV-58 is selective for N- and P/Q-type calcium channels (N- and P/Q; $EC_{50} = 6.8$ and 9.9 μM, respectively) over L-type calcium channels ($EC_{50} > 100$ μM). N- and P/Q-type channels are typically expressed in presynaptic nerve terminals and colocalized with the synaptic vesicle fusion machinery,[35,36] while L-type calcium channels are typically not tightly coupled to transmitter release machinery.[37]

Chemical synthesis of new *R*-roscovitine analogs

Modifications of two of the four side chains of *R*-roscovitine, as well as a review of literature data, provided a first assessment of the structure–activity relationship around the purine core (Fig. 3). Re-

Potential therapeutic impact of novel calcium channel agonists

Because symptomatic strategies that increase transmitter release have emerged as one of the primary treatment strategies for LEMS (especially the potassium channel blocker DAP), the goal is to develop

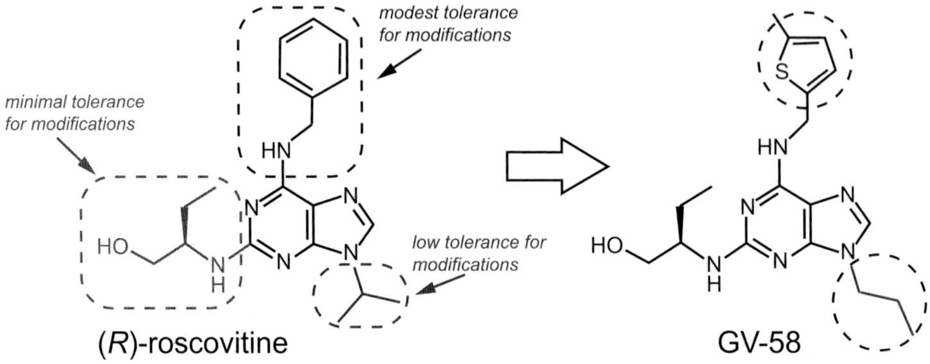

Figure 3. Structure–activity relationship (SAR) summary and comparison of the chemical structure of *R*-roscovitine to GV-58. Dotted-line circles indicate side chains modified in GV-58 (right) compared to (*R*)-roscovitine (left). Adapted from Liang *et al.*[21]

novel calcium channel agonists that may function as alternatives to existing symptomatic treatments for LEMS or represent synergistic agents that may work with existing treatments to reduce neuromuscular weakness.

Further work using animal models of neuromuscular diseases (in particular LEMS) will be required to demonstrate that *in vivo* administration is effective in behavioral assays of muscle weakness. With respect to the potential to act synergistically with existing symptomatic treatments for LEMS, because the current treatment of choice (DAP) broadens the presynaptic action potential, calcium channels will open for a longer period of time during the action potential, and the binding of GV-58 (which is use dependent and occurs to the open configuration of the channel) would be expected to occur more frequently. Therefore, DAP administered in combination with GV-58 may result in a stronger effect that provides an even greater reversal of neuromuscular weakness. The potential for *in vivo* synergistic effects between DAP and GV-58 remains to be tested.

GV-58 represents a first lead structure toward the development of novel calcium channel agonists that have the potential to provide therapeutic benefits to LEMS patients because this disease targets presynaptic calcium channels. While direct therapeutic advantages of a calcium channel agonist for individuals with LEMS is expected based on the etiology of this disease, other neurological diseases affecting the neuromuscular junction may also benefit from a treatment with a selective calcium channel agonist. In particular, congenital myasthenia is a heterogeneous group of inherited disorders caused by mutations in any one of >10 genes that code for synaptic proteins, leading to impaired neuromuscular function.[38–41] In many of these cases, there are few treatment options, and a calcium channel agonist may provide symptomatic relief. Myasthenia gravis is an autoimmune disorder characterized by blockade or loss of acetylcholine receptors at the neuromuscular junction.[42,43] The symptoms of this disorder are often managed using acetylcholinesterase blockers,[13,44,45] but it may be worth examining the effects of calcium channel agonists. Botulism is a rare but serious paralytic illness. Treatment for botulism may take several months, but fatigue may persist for years.[46,47] Botulinum toxin A injections (Botox®) for therapeutic and cosmetic purposes carry a risk of complications, in particular after repeated high-dose injections,[48] and for patients with neurological disorders.[49] At least in some of these cases, a calcium channel agonist may provide symptomatic relief.

Novel *R*-roscovitine analogs as useful experimental tool compounds

Historically, calcium channel gating modifiers have been valuable experimental tools. Because voltage-gated calcium channels have a relatively small conductance and brief mean open time, single channel gating has been relatively difficult to study in detail without the aid of gating modifiers. Furthermore, studies of physiological effects of calcium channels can be aided by the use of gating modifiers. Relatively few calcium channel agonists have been identified (e.g., BayK 8644 and FPL 64176), and those that have been developed only bind selectively to L-type calcium channels.[50,51] These L-type agonists have provided an experimental opportunity to increase mean open time for L-type calcium channels. With this tool, investigators have been better able to determine conductance in physiological calcium concentrations,[52] test for a role of L-type channels in the regulation of transmitter release at synapses,[53–55] study the structural motifs within the L-type calcium channel that regulate gating,[56–58] study the influence of ion permeation on gating,[59] and examine cell signaling that employs L-type calcium channels,[60] among many other experimental uses. The development of novel calcium agonists for N- and P/Q-type channels would provide an opportunity to study these important transmitter-regulating calcium channel subtypes in ways that have only been available previously for the study of L-type channels.

In summary, selective calcium channel agonists have great potential to provide benefits for a wide range of diseases and adverse conditions that are associated with impaired neuromuscular transmission and to advance basic science understanding of the calcium channel types that control transmitter release. *R*-Roscovitine analogs like GV-58 represent the first in a new class of compounds that target selectively the N- and P/Q-type calcium channels expressed selectively at nerve terminals.[61]

Conflicts of interest

The authors declare no conflicts of interest.

References

1. Lambert, E.H., L.M. Eaton & E.D. Rooke. 1956. Defect of neuromuscular conduction associated with malignant neoplasm. *Am. J. Physiol.* **187:** 612–613.
2. Titulaer, M.J., B. Lang & J.J. Verschuuren. 2011. Lambert–Eaton myasthenic syndrome: from clinical characteristics to therapeutic strategies. *Lancet Neurol.* **10:** 1098–1107.
3. Payne, M., P. Bradbury, B. Lang, *et al.* 2011. Prospective study into the incidence of Lambert Eaton myasthenic syndrome in small cell lung cancer. *J. Thorac. Oncol.* **5:** 34–8.
4. Gilhus, N.E. 2012. Myasthenia and the neuromuscular junction. *Curr. Opin. Neurol.* **25:** 523–529.
5. Vincent, A., B. Lang & J. Newsom-Davis. 1989. Autoimmunity to the voltage-gated calcium channel underlies the Lambert–Eaton myasthenic syndrome, a paraneoplastic disorder. *Trends Neurosci.* **12:** 496–502.
6. Nagel, A., A.G. Engel, B. Lang, *et al.* 1988. Lambert–Eaton myasthenic syndrome IgG depletes presynaptic membrane active zone particles by antigenic modulation. *Ann. Neurol.* **24:** 552–558.
7. Meriney, S.D., S.C. Hulsizer, V.A. Lennon & A.D. Grinnell. 1996. Lambert–Eaton myasthenic syndrome IgG removes multiple types of calcium channels from a human small cell lung cancer cell line. *Ann. Neurol.* **40:** 739–749.

8. Abicht, A. & H. Lochmuller. 2002. What's in the serum of seronegative MG and LEMS? *Neurology* **59:** 1672–1673.
9. Raymond, C., D. Walker, D. Bichet, *et al.* 1999. Antibodies against the beta subunit of voltage-dependent calcium channels in Lambert–Eaton myasthenic syndrome. *Neuroscience* **90:** 269–277.
10. Takamori, M., K. Komai & K. Iwasa. 2000. Antibodies to calcium channel and synaptotagmin in Lambert–Eaton myasthenic syndrome. *Am. J. Med. Sci.* **319:** 204–208.
11. Flink, M.T. & W.D. Atchison. 2002. Passive transfer of Lambert–Eaton syndrome to mice induced dihydropyridine sensitivity of neuromuscular transmission. *J. Physiol.* **543:** 567–576.
12. Smith, D.O., M.W. Conklin, P.J. Jensen & W.D. Atchison. 1995. Decreased calcium currents in motor nerve terminals of mice with Lambert–Eaton myasthenic syndrome. *J. Physiol.* **487:** 115–123.
13. Skeie, G.O., S. Apostolski, A. Evoli, *et al.*, European Federation of Neurological Societies. 2010. Guidelines for treatment of autoimmune neuromuscular transmission disorders. *Eur. J. Neurol.* **17:** 893–902.
14. Verschuuren, J.J., P.W. Wirtz, M.J. Titulaer, *et al.* 2006. Available treatment options for the management of Lambert–Eaton myasthenic syndrome. *Expert Opin. Pharmacother.* **7:** 1323–1336.
15. Wirtz, P.W., J.J. Verschuuren, J.G. van Dijk, *et al.* 2009. Efficacy of 3,4-diaminopyridine and pyridostigmine in the treatment of Lambert–Eaton myasthenic syndrome: a randomized, double-blind, placebo-controlled, crossover study. *Clin. Pharmacol. Ther.* **86:** 44–48.
16. Oh, S.J., G.G. Claussen, Y. Hatanaka & M.B. Morgan. 2009. 3,4-Diaminopyridine is more effective than placebo in a randomized, double-blind, cross-over drug study in LEMS. *Muscle Nerve* **40:** 795–800.
17. Sanders, D.B., J.M. Massey, L.L. Sanders & L.J. Edwards. 2000. A randomized trial of 3,4-diaminopyridine in Lambert–Eaton myasthenic syndrome. *Neurology* **54:** 603–607.
18. Miralles, F. & C. Solsona. 1998. 3,4diaminopyridine-induced impairment in frog motor nerve terminal response to high frequency stimulation. *Brain Res.* **789:** 239–244.
19. Thomsen, R.H. & D.F. Wilson. 1983. Effects of 4-aminopyridine and 3,4diaminopyridine on transmitter release at the neuromuscular junction. *J. Pharmacol. Exp. Ther.* **227:** 260–265.
20. Tarr, T.B., W. Malick, M. Liang, *et al.* 2012. *Evaluation of a Novel Calcium Channel Agonist for Potential Therapeutic Activity in LEMS and other Neuromuscular Diseases.* Program No. 653.31. 2012 Neuroscience Meeting Planner. Society for Neuroscience. New Orleans, LA, 2012. Online.
21. Liang, M., T.B. Tarr, K. Bravo-Altamirano, *et al.* 2012. Synthesis and biological evaluation of a new calcium channel agonist. *ACS Med. Chem. Lett.* **3:** 985–990.
22. Paglini, G. & A. Caceres. 2001. The role of the Cdk5–p35 kinase in neuronal development. *Eur. J. Biochem.* **268:** 1528–1533.
23. Cheng, K. & N.Y. Ip. 2003. Cdk5: a new player at synapses. *NeuroSignals* **12:** 180–190.

24. Kesavapany, S., B.S. Li & H.C. Pant. 2003. Cyclin-dependent kinase 5 in neurofilament function and regulation. *NeuroSignals* **12:** 252–264.

25. Smith, D. 2003. Cdk5 in neuroskeletal dynamics. *NeuroSignals* **12:** 239–251.

26. Shelton, S.B. & G.V. Johnson. 2004. Cyclin-dependent kinase-5 in neurodegeneration. *J. Neurochem.* **88:** 1313–1326.

27. Murray, A.W. 2004. Recycling the cell cycle: cyclins revisited. *Cell* **116:** 221–234.

28. Monaco, E.A. & M.L. Vallano. 2003. Cyclin-dependent kinase inhibitors: cancer killers to neuronal guardians. *Curr. Med. Chem.* **10:** 367–379.

29. Yan, Z., P. Chi, J.A. Bibb, *et al.* 2002. Roscovitine: a novel regulator of P/Q-type calcium channels and transmitter release in central neurons. *J. Physiol.* **540:** 761–770.

30. Buraei, Z., M. Anghelescu & K.S. Elmslie. 2005. Slowed N-type calcium channel (CaV2.2) deactivation by the cyclin-dependent kinase inhibitor roscovitine. *Biophys J.* **89:** 1681–1691.

31. Cho, S. & S.D. Meriney. 2006. The effects of presynaptic calcium channel modulation by roscovitine on transmitter release at the adult frog neuromuscular junction. *Eur. J. Neurosci.* **23:** 3200–3208.

32. Tomizawa, K., J. Ohta, M. Matsushita, *et al.* 2002. Cdk5/p35 regulates neurotransmitter release through phosphorylation and downregulation of P/Q-type voltage-dependent calcium channel activity. *J. Neurosci.* **22:** 2590–2597.

33. Buraei, Z., G. Schofield & K.S. Elmslie. 2007. Roscovitine differentially affects CaV2 and Kv channels by binding to the open state. *Neuropharmacology* **52:** 883–894.

34. DeStefino, N.R., A.A. Pilato, M. Dittrich, *et al.* 2010. (R)-Roscovitine prolongs the mean open time of unitary N-type calcium channel currents. *Neuroscience* **167:** 838–849.

35. Protti, D.A., R. Reisin, T.A. Mackinley & O.D. Uchitel. 1996. Calcium channel blockers and transmitter release at the normal human neuromuscular junction. *Neurology* **46:** 1391–1396.

36. Urbano, F.J., M.R. Pagani & O.D. Uchitel. 2008. Calcium channels, neuromuscular synaptic transmission and neurological diseases. *J. Neuroimmunol.* **201–202:** 136–144.

37. Sheng, Z.H., R.E. Westenbroek & W.A. Catterall. 1998. Physical link and functional coupling of presynaptic calcium channels and the synaptic vesicle docking/fusion machinery. *J. Bioenerg. Biomembr.* **30:** 335–345.

38. Palace, J., C.M. Wiles & J. Newsom-Davis. 1991. 3,4-Diaminopyridine in the treatment of congenital (hereditary) myasthenia. *J. Neurol. Neurosurg. Psychiatr.* **54:** 1069–1072.

39. Harper, C.M. 2004. Congenital myasthenic syndromes. *Semin. Neurol.* **24:** 111–123.

40. Pelufo-Pellicer, A., E. Monte-Boquet, E. Romá-Sánchez, *et al.* 2006. Fetal exposure to 3,4-diaminopyridine in a pregnant woman with congenital myasthenia syndrome. *Ann. Pharmacother.* **40:** 762–766.

41. Engel, A.G., X.M. Shen, D. Selcen & S.M. Sine. 2009. What have we learned from the congenital myasthenic syndromes. *J. Mol. Neurosci.* **40:** 143–153.

42. Patrick, J. & J. Lindstrom. 1973. Autoimmune response to acetylcholine receptors. *Science* **180:** 871–872.

43. Meriggioli, M.N. & D.B. Sanders. 2009. Autoimmune myasthenia gravis: emerging clinical and biological heterogeneity. *Lancet Neurol.* **8:** 475–490.

44. Gilhus, N.E., J.F. Owe, J.M. Hoff, *et al.* 2011. Myasthenia gravis: a review of available treatment approaches. *Autoimmune Dis.* **2011:** 1–6.

45. Sathasivam, S. 2011. Current and emerging treatments for the management of myasthenia gravis. *Ther. Clin. Risk Manag.* **7:** 313–23.

46. Mann, J.M., S. Martin, R. Hoffman & S. Marrazzo. 1981. Patient recovery from type A botulism: morbidity assessment following a large outbreak. *Am. J. Public Health* **1:** 266–269.

47. Wilcox, P., G. Andolfatto, M.S. Fairbarn & R.L Pardy. 1989. Long-term follow-up of symptoms, pulmonary function, respiratory muscle strength, and exercise performance after botulism. *Am. Rev. Respir. Dis.* **139:** 157–163.

48. Crowner, B.E., D. Torres-Russotto, A.R, Carter & B.A. Racette. 2010. Systemic weakness after therapeutic injections of botulinum toxin a: a case series and review of the literature. *Clin. Neuropharmacol.* **33:** 243–247.

49. Dressler, D. 2010. Subclinical myasthenia gravis causing increased sensitivity to botulinum toxin therapy. *J. Neural. Transm.* **117:** 1293–1294.

50. Zheng, W., D. Rampe & D.J. Triggle. 1991. Pharmacological, radio ligand binding, and electrophysiological characteristics of FPL 64176, a novel nondihydropyridine Ca^{2+} channel activator, in cardiac and vascular preparations. *Mol. Pharmacol.* **40:** 734–741.

51. Hess, P., J.B. Lansman & R.W. Tsien. 1984. Different modes of Ca channel gating behavior favoured by dihydropyridine Ca agonists and antagonists. *Nature* **311:** 538–544.

52. Church, P.J. & E.F. Stanley. 1996. Single L-type calcium channel conductance with physiological levels of calcium in chick ciliary ganglion neurons. *J. Physiol.* **496:** 59–68.

53. Yu, C., M. Jia, M. Litzinger & P.G. Nelson. 1988. Calcium agonist (BayK 8644) augments voltage-sensitive calcium currents but not synaptic transmission in cultured mouse spinal cord neurons. *Exp. Brain Res.* **71:** 467–474.

54. Jensen, K., M.S. Jensen & J.D. Lambert. 1999. Role of presynaptic L-type Ca^{2+} channels in GABAergic synaptic transmission in cultured hippocampal neurons. *J. Neurophysiol.* **81:** 1225–1230.

55. Holmgaard, K., K. Jensen & J.D. Lambert. 2009. Imaging of Ca^{2+} responses mediated by presynaptic L-type channels on GABAergic boutons of cultured hippocampal neurons. *Brain Res.* **1249:** 79–90.

56. Mitterdorfer, J., Z. Wang, M.J. Sinnegger, *et al.* 1996. Two amino acid residues in the IIIS5 segment of L-type calcium channels differentially contribute to 1,4-dihydropyridine sensitivity. *J. Biol. Chem.* **271:** 30330–30335.

57. Grabner, M., Z. Wang, S. Hering, *et al.* 1996. Transfer of 1,4-dihydropyridine sensitivity from L-type to class A (BI) calcium channels. *Neuron* **16:** 207–218.

58. Erxleben, C., C. Gomez-Alegria, T. Darden, *et al.* 2003. Modulation of cardiac Ca(V)1.2 channels by dihydropyridine and phosphatase inhibitor requires Ser-1142 in the domain III pore loop. *Proc. Natl. Acad. Sci. USA* **100:** 2929–2934.

59. Hui, K., P. Gardzinski, H.S. Sun, *et al.* 2005. Permeable ions differentially affect gating kinetics and unitary conductance of L-type calcium channels. *Biochem Biophys. Res. Commun.* **338:** 783–792.

60. Katoh, H., K. Schlotthauer & D.M. Bers. 2000. Transmission of information from cardiac dihydropyridine receptor to ryanodine receptor: evidence from BayK 8644 effects on resting Ca(2+) sparks. *Circ. Res.* **87:** 106–111.

61. Evans, R.M. & G.W. Zamponi. 2006. Presynaptic Ca^{2+} channels—integration centers for neuronal signaling pathways. *Trends Neurosci.* **29:** 617–624.

Ann. N.Y. Acad. Sci. ISSN 0077-8923

Thymus pathology observed in the MGTX trial

Alexander Marx,[1][*] Frederik Pfister,[1][*] Berthold Schalke,[3] Wilfred Nix,[4] and Philipp Ströbel[1,2]

[1]Institute of Pathology, University Medical Center Mannheim, University of Heidelberg, Mannheim, Germany. [2]Institute of Pathology, University of Göttingen, Göttingen, Germany. [3]Neurology Clinic, University of Regensburg, Regensburg, Germany. [4]Neurology Clinic, University of Mainz, Mainz, Germany

Address for correspondence: Alexander Marx, M.D., Institute of Pathology, University Medical Center Mannheim, University of Heidelberg, Theodor-Kutzer-Ufer 1-3, D-68167 Mannheim, Germany. alexander.marx@umm.de

The MGTX trial is the first prospective, randomized clinical trial that aims to evaluate the impact of extended transsternal thymectomy on myasthenic symptoms, prednisone requirements, and quality of life in patients with non-thymomatous, anti-acetylcholine receptor autoantibody-positive myasthenia gravis (MG). Here, we give an overview of the rationale of thymectomy and the standardized macroscopic and histopathological work-up of thymectomy specimens as fixed in MGTX standard operating procedures, including the grading of thymic lymphofollicular hyperplasia and the morphometric strategy to assess thymic involution.

Keywords: thymectomy; thymitis; thymic atrophy; involution; morphometry; CD23

Historic overview on thymectomy in myasthenia gravis and the MGTX trial

Improvement of myasthenic symptoms following thymectomy was first reported in 1911 by Ferdinand Sauerbruch who removed the thymus in a young female with hyperthyroidism and myasthenia gravis (MG).[1] However, it was Blalock who first published results of a series of thymectomies that were specifically performed to treat MG, revealed clinical benefit in a large subset of patients, and initiated the world-wide popularization of thymic surgery that began in 1940.[2] Many subsequent studies continued to report on the amelioration of MG symptoms following thymectomy in some but not all patients (reviewed by Sonnett[3]), even after the introduction of various highly effective antimyasthenic agents like cholinesterase inhibitors,[4] corticosteroids,[5] azathioprine,[6] and intravenous immunoglobulins.[7]

The patients who profit most from thymectomy apparently are those who suffer from generalized early-onset MG (EOMG).[3,8,9] By definition, these nonthymomatous patients have serum anti-acetylcholinereceptor (AChR) autoantibodies and

usually show thymic lymphofollicular hyperplasia and a strong bias for female gender and a high-risk HLA haplotype.[10–12] Whether an age threshold of 50 or 60 years is appropriate to delineate EOMG from late-onset MG (LOMG) patients is currently an unsettled question.[13–15] By contrast, thymectomy is of no or little clinical benefit in the vast majority of patients with LOMG and anti-MuSK autoantibody-positive MG (with few exceptions[16–18]), and benefit is highly variable and somewhat controversial in thymoma-associated MG.[8,9,19–28] The lack of a beneficial effect of thymectomy is associated with a largely normal-for-age histology of the thymus in LOMG and MuSK[+] MG, while the remnant thymus in cases of myasthenic thymomas shows thymic lymphofollicular hyperplasia (TFH) in up to 30% of cases; however, it is not known whether the degree of TFH in the remnant thymus is related to the variable post-surgery course of thymoma-associated MG.[19,29–33]

The current clinical rationale for thymectomy in EOMG is strongly supported by experimental evidence. Available data suggest that EOMG apparently begins in the thymus by so far enigmatic triggers and is maintained there by an ongoing pathological immune reaction. This pathological immune reaction involves peptides derived from single AChR

---

[*]These authors contributed equally

doi: 10.1111/j.1749-6632.2012.06799.x

subunits that are expressed by medullary thymic epithelial cells and likely prime autoreactive T cells (that are known to occur in the normal T cell repertoire[34,35]); autoantibodies that attack fully developed, pentameric AChRs expressed on the surface of thymic myoid cells; and immune complexes that activate antigen presenting cells, drive the development of lymphoid follicles with germinal centers, and contribute to autoantibody diversification and the generation of long-lived plasma cells inside and—later on—outside the thymus ("intrathymic pathogenesis").[11,36–38]

Considering this biological background of EOMG and the known wide-spread distribution of inflamed thymic tissue across the cervical and mediastinal region in many EOMG patients, researchers agreed that early[39] and total ("maximal") transcervical–transsternal thymectomy[28] would be desirable.[3,40,41] However, practical considerations that are mainly centered on the prevention of potential severe side effects of total thymectomy (like phrenic nerve injury) have made the slightly less invasive "extended thymectomy" the most feasible surgical technique in EOMG,[3] though with an ongoing debate whether the standard transsternal approach or recently introduced minimally invasive procedures yield better results for MG outcome.[3,42–44]

Despite the long history of thymectomy and its popularity as a treatment facet of EOMG, formal evidence is lacking that surgery adds significantly to the benefits of properly performed treatment with corticosteroids and immunosuppressive agents. This is unsatisfactory considering the poorly understood role of the thymus in the elderly, the limited knowledge about long-term effects of thymectomy on immune reactions against infectious or tumor-related antigens, and the indispensible role of the thymus for the reestablishment of T cell immunity and immunological competence after chemotherapy and bone marrow transplantation.[45,46]

To resolve the role of thymectomy in MG management, the thymectomy trial for nonthymomatous MG patients receiving prednisone (MGTX) was designed as an NINDS cooperative multinational, multicenter, two-arm trial.[47] It aims to determine whether extended transsternal thymectomy (T-3b according to the Myathenia Gravis Foundation of America) plus prednisone compared to prednisone

alone results in a greater improvement in MG weakness, a lower total dose of prednisone, and an enhanced quality of life by reducing adverse events and symptoms.[48,49] Since the degree of preoperative thymic pathology is a likely variable that might influence the impact of thymectomy on the outcome of MG,[40,50] histological evaluation of the thymectomy specimens is an integral part of the MGTX trial.

After having collected about half of the intended specimens, we aim here to give an interim report about the quality of the received material; the feasibility of the formalin-fixed, paraffin-embedded material for special examinations, such as immunohistochemistry, semiquantative grading of lymphofollicular hyperplasia, and morphometric quantification of thymic involution; and the broad spectrum of histological findings encountered so far that apparently reflect variable use of prednisone or heterogeneous responsiveness to prednisone, and suggest that the correlation of pathological alterations with parameters of clinical interest can be done after completion of the recruitment of patients and analysis of their thymectomy specimens.

Aims of the histological evaluation and preliminary study population

The original aims of the pathology study within the MGTX were to assess the degree of TFH; the extent of overall atrophy of thymic parenchyma; the degree of cortical involution in the formalin fixed, paraffin-embedded material of an expected 100 thymectomy cases obtained within the MGTX trial from all over the world; and to correlate morphological findings with various clinical features by multivariate analysis at the end of the trial. However, we obtained only 51 cases so far: one cohort of 17 cases in 2008 and another cohort of 34 cases in April 2012. Both cohorts shared a high percentage of females (76%) in good agreement with epidemiological data in different ethnicities.[10,15,40,51–53] In the two cohorts, the percentages of patients over 40 years of age were identical (35%), while those of patients over 50 were slightly different (12 and 21%, respectively), as were mean ages (33 years, range 18–57 years in the first, 37 years, range 18–63 years, in the second cohort). These basic epidemiological observations argue against a major recruitment bias during the period in which the first half of the intended patients were recruited (not excluding a recruitment bias as far as the whole population of MG patients is concerned). Therefore, the two cohorts will henceforth be considered together. Although the preliminary morphological analysis of this low number of cases is clearly inadequate to draw any conclusions about the trial outcome, the observations made so far served to confirm the adequacy and usefulness of the pathology-related standard operating procedures that we describe next.

Pathology-related standard operating procedures

Sampling strategy and tissue quality

Work-up of the thymectomy specimen followed a standardized protocol that was approved by the MGTX advisory committee.[49] Immediately (within 10 min) after extended transsternal thymectomy[3] six blocks of fresh material from different thymic regions and one block of thymus-free mediastinal adipose tissue were cryopreserved in liquid nitrogen for subsequent biomarker and molecular studies. The remaining material was fixed for 24 ± 2 h in 10% neutral buffered formalin, and a minimum of 12 blocks of at least 1 cm diameter from various defined regions were paraffin embedded (including a central horizontal plain that was embedded completely). This standard operating procedure (SOP) has continuously guaranteed high tissue quality of paraffin-embedded material, since excellent or good quality material was detected by histological analysis in 87% of the cases. In about 10% of cases minor fixation artifacts were encountered, but only one recent case was so poorly preserved that histological and immunohistochemical evaluation of follicular hyperplasia was not possible.

Morphometry and immunohistochemistry

The pathology-related protocol of the MGTX trial suggests to apply morphometry to H&E-stained sections to quantify content of thymic parenchyma in relation to interstitial fat, and cortical compared to medullary compartments. In addition to H&E-based morphometry, the protocol also suggests to perform immunoperoxidase-based immunohistochemistry using 4 μm–thick sections of paraffin-embedded material for the detection of follicular dendritic cells (CD23, see below) and germinal center B cells (CD10, not shown) as surrogate markers of early and late germinal center development, respectively.[37,54,55] Morphometric analysis was per-

formed using the cellF image analysis software (Olympus, Münster, Germany). Analyses were performed blinded to epidemiological and clinical details, including duration and dosage of preoperative prednisone treatment.

A grading system of thymic lymphofollicular hyperplasia for tentative testing

In order to allow for semiquantitative assessment and description of thymic lymphofollicular hyperplasia (TFH), the MGTX protocol proposes the 4-tiered scoring system illustrated in Fig. 1A–C for tentative testing. The system requires H&E-stained routinely processed sections (Fig. 1A) and the enumeration of low power fields (LPFs, at × 50 magnification) that either contain or do not contain lymphoid follicles (with and without obvious germinal centers, GCs, Fig. 1B). In analogy to the enumeration and quantification of mitoses in many cancers, we tentatively propose to assess follicle content as the percentage of follicle-positive LPFs per 20 LPFs and assign a given case to one of the TFH grades I to III that cover the 1–33%, 34–66%, and 67–100% ranges, respectively (Fig. 1C). Grade IV TFH is diagnosed if more than three follicles per any LPF are detected. Grade IV TFH can occur against a background of focal (grade I and II) or diffuse (grade III) TFH. This heterogeneity among TFH grade IV cases may be expressed as TFH grades I/IV, II/IV, and III/IV. We have used this scheme for years in our daily clinical practice after we observed the following meaningful correlations: absence of lymphoid follicles and TFH grade 1 can be observed in normal thymic tissue of children and adults without obvious association with autoimmune or other diseases;[56,57] TFH grades II and III are characteristic of EOMG but can rarely occur in nonmyasthenic patients with autoimmune disease like Sjögren's disease, hyperthyroidism, lupus eythematosus, systemic sclerosis, and rheumatoid arthritis;[50,57–59] TFG grade IV is virtually pathognomonic for EOMG, particularly when it occurs as a focal phenomenon;[31] and the TFH grading rules outlined above are also applicable to standard thymus histological preparations outside clinical studies where less than 20 LPFs of tissue are often available.

The above system was easily applicable to the specimens of 50 out of the 51 MGTX patients studied so far and revealed that only 25% of patients showed thymic alterations that are characteristic

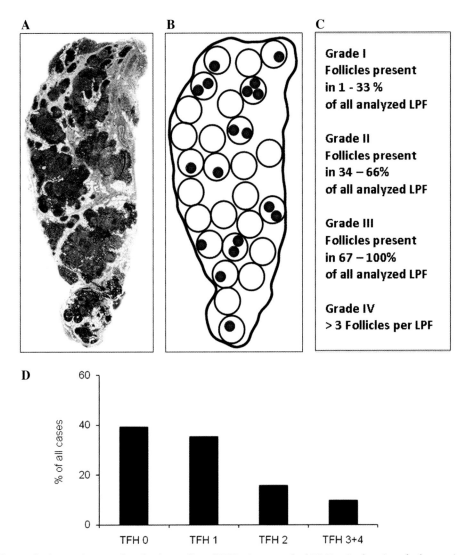

Figure 1. Standard operating procedure for the grading of TFH using a standard H&E-stained section of a thymus tissue sample and testing in a pilot series of cases. Presence of lymphoid follicles is analyzed in randomly selected low-power fields covering areas with lymphoid parenchyma (LPF, ×50 magnification) (A). Schematic illustration of the analysis of LPFs (black circles) and lymphoid follicles (red dots). In this particular case, 12 of 27 LPFs contain 1 to 3 lymphoid follicles (44%) (B). According to the grading system shown in C, this case was graded as TFH grade II. D shows the distribution of TFH grades in the first 50 patients with adequate tissue studied so far. TFH0: no TFH.

of EOMG—that is, who show TFH grade II-IV (Fig. 1D). Most of the cases showed mild or no lympho-follicular hyperplasia. Considering the fact that we are still blind to any clinical details, we have no firm conclusion that can be drawn so far from these preliminary observations. In theory, the relatively low percentage of higher grade TFH in the current series could hint to very early time points of thymectomy during the natural course of MG.[54] Alternatively, and maybe more likely in light of the substantial thymic involution encountered so far (see below), extensive preoperative prednisone treatment could have played a role.[60] Therefore, it will be interesting to see after the end of the trial, whether differences for TFH grades between the two available cohorts and between these and the future cohort are related to differences of average age, to different percentages of patients over 50 years of age, and different preoperative periods of prednisone treatment or combinations thereof.

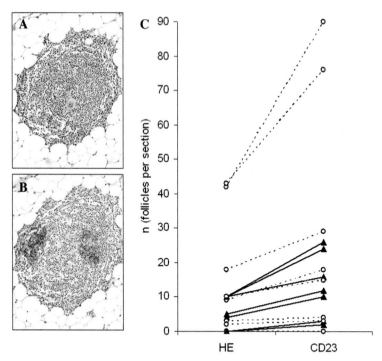

Figure 2. Impact of CD23 staining on TFH grading compared to conventional TFH grading, as based on H&E histology assessed in the first 17 cases received in 2008. H&E-stained, severely atrophic (cortex-deficient) thymic lobule without recognizable follicles or germinal centers (A). Two networks of CD23-positive follicular dendritic cells (immunoperoxidase; x 100), suggesting occurrence of either early lymphoid follicle development or—more likely in conjunction with thymic atrophy—remnant follicles after prednisone-induced involution (B). Counting of H&E-stained compared to CD23-positive follicles increased the yield of follicle counts per section and increased the TFH grade in seven cases (solid lines, triangles), but not in the other 10 cases (broken line). Each line represents one patient (C). Which approach (H&E or anti-CD23 staining) is clinically more meaningful is currently unknown.

Grading of thymic follicular hyperplasia based on H&E staining versus immunohistochemical detection of follicles

The most relevant clinical strategy to gauge the degree of thymic follicular hyperplasia as a candidate biomarker for the postoperative management of MG is unknown. To better understand whether immunohistochemical detection of lymphoid follicles with and without germinal centers will only facilitate TFH grading or will change the TFH grade by substantially increasing the sensitivity of follicle detection, the MGTX protocol suggests the comparison of TFH grading strategies. These strategies are alternatively based on H&E histology or on the immunohistochemical detection of either CD23 in follicular dendritic cells or CD10 (not shown) on germinal center B cells, respectively. Our preliminary observations made in the cohort of specimens received in 2008 ($n = 17$) showed that anti-CD23 immunostaining increased the numbers of detected follicles in most cases (> 80%) when compared to H&E his-

tology in agreement with a limited historic study.[54] Furthermore, the higher sensitivity of immunohistochemistry compared to H&E histology to detect lymphoid follicles, had an impact on TFH grading: the CD23-based TFH immune-grade was one grade higher than the H&E-based TFH grade in a substantial proportion (about 40%) of cases (Fig. 2). To substantiate or refute the relevance of this preliminary observation, independent confirmation in other cohorts of thymectomy specimens and correlation with clinical parameters will be needed.

Morphometry of thymus parenchyma and cortical versus medullary compartments

As a quality control of our morphometric strategy, we measured the extent of overall thymic atrophy by semiautomatic image analysis that separated thymic parenchyma from intervening and surrounding adipose tissue. This is shown for two patients with highly disparate "fatty involution" in Fig. 3A and B. In addition, we quantified the percentage of cortical

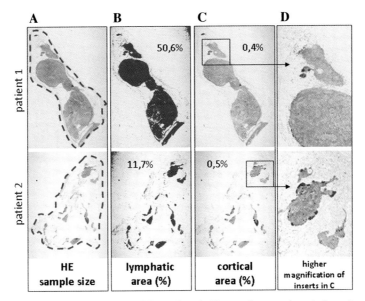

Figure 3. Illustration of the quantification process of thymic lymphoid parenchyma and cortical area in representative samples of two patients. In standard H&E-stained sections, total tissue size was measured (A, red dotted line). Next, the lymphatic tissue component was quantified as the percentage of total tissue sample by an imaging analysis system after manual adaption of the staining intensity recognition threshold. In B, the threshold was adapted to the total lymphatic area with suppression of the surrounding fat and connective tissue. In C, the threshold was adapted to optimize distinction between dark-staining cortical and light-staining medullary regions. D shows detailed pictures of the inset in C.

areas in relation to the whole thymic parenchyma by manually adjusting the threshold of the imaging system to distinguish dark-staining cortical areas from light-grey medullary regions (Fig. 3C and D). By this techniques, we show that the overall parenchymal content with an average of 28% and cortical involution were well within the range of age-adjusted standard values published previously for nonmyasthenic thymuses (Fig. 4A and B).[31] Even though we are still blind to all clinical parameters, the impact of preoperative immunosuppression on histology could not be overlooked, since it was particularly striking in the youngest patients (18–21 years, $n =$ 9), who showed a broad spectrum of thymic atrophy and cortical involution: Using age-adjusted normal values for nonmyasthenic normal thymuses,[31] the observed histologies were either adequate for age ($n = 2$), more adequate for 40 years of age ($n = 2$) or reflecting massive atrophy as it is normally encountered in people over 60 ($n = 5$).

Perspectives

The current pilot study of the first 51 out of an expected 100 cases of thymectomy specimens reports on work in progress and was undertaken to test the adequacy of the standard operating procedures chosen by the MGTX trial protocol but does not, however, allow any conclusions to be drawn about the outcome of the MGTX trial. Nevertheless, these preliminary observations suggest that the material retrieved within the MGTX trial is mostly well suited for the planned biomarker studies—provided that the quality of the paraffin-embedded material is representative of the cryomaterial. Nevertheless, considering the occurrence of rare cases with poor tissue preservation and the high degree of heterogeneity for tissue content and thymic follicular hyperplasia, we propose that thorough preanalytical quality control of the cryomaterial by histology will be indispensible to achieve meaningful molecular results. The introduced strategy to grade TFH and the derived grading system is currently tentative for testing, that is, it will need to be evaluated and validated by correlation with clinical data (including MG outcome and duration and intensity of preoperative immunosuppression) that will become available once recruitment and follow-up period of the MGTX trial will be finished. Specifically, the mainly arbitrary thresholds (33%, 66%) will need reconsideration. Whether H&E-based grading of TFH,

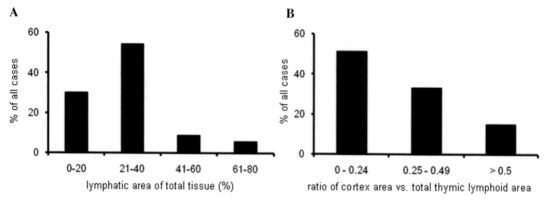

Figure 4. Pilot study of quantitative, semiautomatic measurement of thymic lymphoid parenchyma and cortical areas in the patients studied to date using the method illustrated in Fig. 3. Percentage of thymic lymphoid parenchyma ("lymphatic area of total tissue"; A) and the proportion of cortical area in relation to thymic parenchyma ("ratio of cortex area vs. total thymic lymphoid area"; B).

grading based on the counting of CD23-positive follicular dendritic networks (of either early or involuted follicles), or the enumeration of CD10-positive mature and active germinal centers will yield more clinically important information is currently unknown. An answer to these open questions will likely shed light on the currently favored two-step model of intrathymic pathogenesis of anti-AChR-positive nonthymomatous MG.[11,37] Considering the heterogeneity of our preliminary histological observations even within the same age groups, we will be excited to see whether meaningful correlations between preoperative histological parameters and patient outcome for myasthenic symptoms can be established after completion of the MGTX trial.

Acknowledgments

This work was supported by a grant from the Myasthenia Gravis Foundation of America to A.M. and P.S.; myasthenia gravis–related work in the Marx laboratory is supported by the German Ministry of Education and Research (BMBF) (Grant 01DL12027).

Conflicts of interest

The authors declare no conflicts of interest.

References

1. Sauerbruch, E.F. 1913. Thymektomie bei einem Fall von Morbus Basedow mit Myasthenie. *Mitt. Grenzgeb. Med. Chir.* **25:** 746–765.
2. Blalock, A. 1944. Thymectomy in the treatment of myasthenia gravis: report of twenty cases. *J. Thorac. Surg.* **13:** 316–339.
3. Sonett, J.R. & A. Jaretzki, 3rd. 2008. Thymectomy for nonthymomatous myasthenia gravis: a critical analysis. *Ann. N. Y. Acad. Sci.* **1132:** 315–328.
4. Walker, M.B. 1934. Treatment of Myasthenia gravis with Physostigmine. *Lancet* I: 1200–1201.
5. Grob, D. & T. Namba. 1966. Corticotropin in generalized myasthenia gravis. Effect of short, intensive courses. *JAMA* **198:** 703–707.
6. Mertens, H.G., F. Balzereit & M. Leipert. 1969. The treatment of severe myasthenia gravis with immunosuppressive agents. *Eur. Neurol.* **2:** 321–339.
7. Arsura, E.L. *et al.* 1986. High-dose intravenous immunoglobulin in the management of myasthenia gravis. *Archive. Inter. Med.* **146:** 1365–1368.
8. Skeie, G.O. *et al.* 2010. Guidelines for treatment of autoimmune neuromuscular transmission disorders. *Eur. J. Neurol.* **17:** 893–902.
9. Gilhus, N.E. *et al.* 2011. Myasthenia gravis: a review of available treatment approaches. *Autoimmun. Dis.* **2011:** 847393.
10. Drachman, D.B. 1994. Myasthenia gravis. *N. Engl. J. Med.* **330:** 1797–1810.
11. Shiono, H. *et al.* 2003. Scenarios for autoimmunization of T and B cells in myasthenia gravis. *Ann. N. Y. Acad. Sci.* **998:** 237–256.
12. Giraud, M., C. Vandiedonck & H.J. Garchon. 2008. Genetic factors in autoimmune myasthenia gravis. *Ann. N. Y. Acad. Sci.* **1132:** 180–192.
13. Aarli, J.A. 2008. Myasthenia gravis in the elderly: is it different? *Ann. N. Y. Acad. Sci.* **1132:** 238–243.
14. Fraisse, T. *et al.* 2007. Myasthenia gravis in the elderly. Diagnosis, comorbidity and course: 45 cases. *Presse. Med.* **36:** 9–14.
15. Pedersen, E.G. *et al.* 2012. Late-onset myasthenia not on the increase: a nationwide register study in Denmark, 1996–2009. *Europ. J. Neurol.* Aug 10. doi:10.1111/j.1468-1331.2012.03850.x [Epub ahead of print]
16. Spengos, K. *et al.* 2008. Dropped head syndrome as prominent clinical feature in MuSK-positive Myasthenia Gravis

with thymus hyperplasia. *Neuromuscular Disord.* **18:** 175–177.

17. Kawaguchi, N. *et al.* 2007. Effects of thymectomy on late-onset myasthenia gravis without thymoma. *Clin. Neurol. Neurosurg.* **109:** 858–861.

18. Tsuchida, M. *et al.* 1999. Efficacy and safety of extended thymectomy for elderly patients with myasthenia gravis. *Ann. Thor. Surg.* **67:** 1563–1567.

19. Romi, F. *et al.* 2002. Thymectomy and anti-muscle autoantibodies in late-onset myasthenia gravis. *Eur. J. Neurol.* **9:** 55–61.

20. Marx, A. *et al.* 2010. Thymoma and paraneoplastic myasthenia gravis. *Autoimmunity* **43:** 413–427.

21. Romi, F. *et al.* 2003. Disease severity and outcome in thymoma myasthenia gravis: a long-term observation study. *Eur. J. Neurol.* **10:** 701–706.

22. de Perrot, M. *et al.* 2002. Prognostic significance of thymomas in patients with myasthenia gravis. *Ann. Thor. Surg.* **74:** 1658–1662.

23. Tsinzerling, N. *et al.* 2007. Myasthenia gravis: a long term follow-up study of Swedish patients with specific reference to thymic histology. *J. Neurol., Neurosurg., Psychiatr.* **78:** 1109–1112.

24. Maggi, L. *et al.* 2008. Thymoma-associated myasthenia gravis: outcome, clinical and pathological correlations in 197 patients on a 20-year experience. *J. Neuroimmunol.* **201–202:** 237–244.

25. Lucchi, M. *et al.* 2009. Association of thymoma and myasthenia gravis: oncological and neurological results of the surgical treatment. *Eur. J. Cardio-Thoracic Surg.* **35:** 812–816; discussion 816.

26. Prokakis, C. *et al.* 2009. Modified maximal thymectomy for myasthenia gravis: effect of maximal resection on late neurologic outcome and predictors of disease remission. *Annal. Thorac. Surg.* **88:** 1638–1645.

27. Hsu, H.S. *et al.* 2006. Thymoma is associated with relapse of symptoms after transsternal thymectomy for myasthenia gravis. *Interact. Cardiovasc. Thorac. Surg.* **5:** 42–46.

28. Jaretzki, A., 3rd *et al.* 1988. "Maximal" thymectomy for myasthenia gravis. Results. *J. Thorac. Cardiovasc. Surg.* **95:** 747–757.

29. Evoli, A. *et al.* 2003. Clinical correlates with anti-MuSK antibodies in generalized seronegative myasthenia gravis. *Brain* **126:** 2304–2311.

30. Leite, M.I. *et al.* 2005. Fewer thymic changes in MuSK antibody-positive than in MuSK antibody-negative MG. *Annal. Neurol.* **57:** 444–448.

31. Strobel, P. *et al.* 2008. The ageing and myasthenic thymus: a morphometric study validating a standard procedure in the histological workup of thymic specimens. *J. Neuroimmunol.* **201–202:** 64–73.

32. Reinhardt, C. & A. Melms. 2000. Normalization of elevated CD4-/CD8- (double-negative) T cells after thymectomy parallels clinical remission in myasthenia gravis associated with thymic hyperplasia but not thymoma. *Annal. Neurol.* **48:** 603–608.

33. Willcox, N. *et al.* 1991. The thymus in seronegative myasthenia gravis patients. *J. Neurol.* **238:** 256–261.

34. Melms, A. *et al.* 1992. T cells from normal and myasthenic individuals recognize the human acetylcholine receptor: heterogeneity of antigenic sites on the alpha-subunit. *Annal. Neurol.* **31:** 311–318.

35. Melms, A. *et al.* 1993. Acetylcholine receptor-specific T cells are present in the normal immune repertoire. A study with recombinant polypeptides of the human acetylcholine receptor alpha-subunit. *Annal. N. Y. Acad. Sci.* **681:** 310–312.

36. Wekerle, H. & U.P. Ketelsen. 1977. Intrathymic pathogenesis and dual genetic control of myasthenia gravis. *Lancet* **1:** 678–680.

37. Leite, M.I. *et al.* 2007. Myasthenia gravis thymus: complement vulnerability of epithelial and myoid cells, complement attack on them, and correlations with autoantibody status. *Am. J. Pathol.* **171:** 893–905.

38. Le Panse, R. *et al.* 2010. Thymic remodeling associated with hyperplasia in myasthenia gravis. *Autoimmunity* **43:** 401–412.

39. Nieto, I.P. *et al.* 1999. Prognostic factors for myasthenia gravis treated by thymectomy: review of 61 cases. *Annal. Thorac. Surg.* **67:** 1568–1571.

40. Genkins, G. *et al.* 1975. Studies in myasthenia gravis: early thymectomy. Electrophysiologic and pathologic correlations. *Am. J. Med.* **58:** 517–524.

41. Ponseti, J.M. *et al.* 2008. Influence of ectopic thymic tissue on clinical outcome following extended thymectomy in generalized seropositive nonthymomatous myasthenia gravis. *Eur. J. Cardio-Thorac. Surg.* **34:** 1062–1067.

42. Ruckert, J.C. *et al.* 2003. Matched-pair comparison of three different approaches for thymectomy in myasthenia gravis. *Surg. Endoscop.* **17:** 711–715.

43. Ruckert, J.C., M. Swierzy & M. Ismail. 2011. Comparison of robotic and nonrobotic thoracoscopic thymectomy: a cohort study. *J. Thorac. Cardiovas. Surg.* **141:** 673–677.

44. Weksler, B. *et al.* 2012. Robot-assisted thymectomy is superior to transsternal thymectomy. *Surg. Endoscop.* **26:** 261–266.

45. Afifi, A. *et al.* 2010. For neonates undergoing cardiac surgery does thymectomy as opposed to thymic preservation have any adverse immunological consequences? *Interact. Cardiovasc. Thorac. Surg.* **11:** 287–291.

46. Miller, J.F. 2011. The golden anniversary of the thymus. Nature reviews. *Immunology* **11:** 489–495.

47. Wolfe, G.I. *et al.* 2003. Development of a thymectomy trial in nonthymomatous myasthenia gravis patients receiving immunosuppressive therapy. *Annal. N. Y. Acad. Sci.* **998:** 473–480.

48. Newsom-Davis, J. *et al.* 2008. Status of the thymectomy trial for nonthymomatous myasthenia gravis patients receiving prednisone. *Annal. N. Y. Acad. Sci.* **1132:** 344–347.

49. Aban, I.B. *et al.* 2008. The MGTX experience: challenges in planning and executing an international, multicenter clinical trial. *J. Neuroimmunol.* **201–202:** 80–84.

50. Mori, T. *et al.* 2007. The distribution of parenchyma, follicles, and lymphocyte subsets in thymus of patients with myasthenia gravis, with special reference to remission after thymectomy. *J. Thorac. Cardiovas. Surg.* **133:** 364–368.

51. Chiu, H.C. *et al.* 1987. Myasthenia gravis: population differences in disease expression and acetylcholine receptor

antibody titers between Chinese and Caucasians. *Neurology* **37:** 1854–1857.

52. Somnier, F.E. 2005. Increasing incidence of late-onset anti-AChR antibody-seropositive myasthenia gravis. *Neurology* **65:** 928–930.

53. Murai, H. *et al.* 2011. Characteristics of myasthenia gravis according to onset-age: Japanese nationwide survey. *J. Neurol. Sci.* **305:** 97–102.

54. Kirchner, T. *et al.* 1986. Immunohistological patterns of non-neoplastic changes in the thymus in Myasthenia gravis. *Virch. Archiv. B, Cell Pathol. include. Molecul. Pathol.* **52:** 237–257.

55. Roxanis, I. *et al.* 2002. Thymic myoid cells and germinal center formation in myasthenia gravis; possible roles in pathogenesis. *J. Neuroimmunol.* **125:** 185–197.

56. Levine, G.D. & J. Rosai. 1978. Thymic hyperplasia and neoplasia: a review of current concepts. *Hum. Pathol.* **9:** 495–515.

57. Okabe, H. 1966. Thymic lymph follicles; a histopathological study of 1,356 autopsy cases. *Acta Pathol. Japonica.* **16:** 109–130.

58. Smith, S.M. & L.J. Ossa-Gomez. 1981. A quantitative histologic comparison of the thymus in 100 healthy and diseased adults. *Am. J. Clin. Pathol.* **76:** 657–665.

59. Ferri, C. *et al.* 2006. Thymus alterations and systemic sclerosis. *Rheumatology* **45:** 72–75.

60. Willcox, N. *et al.* 1989. Variable corticosteroid sensitivity of thymic cortex and medullary peripheral-type lymphoid tissue in myasthenia gravis patients: structural and functional effects. *Qtly. J. Med.* **73:** 1071–1087.

Ann. N.Y. Acad. Sci. ISSN 0077-8923

Biomarker development for myasthenia gravis

Henry J. Kaminski,[1,2] Linda L. Kusner,[2] Gil I. Wolfe,[3] Inmaculada Aban,[4] Greg Minisman,[4] Robin Conwit,[5] and Gary Cutter[4]

Departments of [1]Neurology and [2]Pharmacology and Physiology, George Washington University, Washington, DC. [3]Department of Neurology, University at Buffalo School of Medicine and Biomedical Sciences, The State University of New York, Buffalo, New York. [4]Department of Biostatistics, University of Alabama School of Public Health, Birmingham, Alabama. [5]Division of Extramural Research, NIH/NINDS, Bethesda, Maryland

Address for correspondence: Henry J. Kaminski, M.D., Department of Neurology, George Washington University, 2150 Pennsylvania Avenue, Washington DC 20037. HKaminski@mfa.gwu.edu

Biomarkers are defined as characteristics (e.g., proteins, RNA, single nucleotide polymorphisms, imaging) that are objectively measured and evaluated as indicators of pathogenic processes or pharmacologic responses to therapeutic intervention. Biomarkers are important in clinical trials where the robust biomarker reflects the underlying disease process in a sensitive and reliable manner. For myasthenia gravis (MG), acetylcholine receptor and muscle-specific kinase antibodies, as well as single-fiber electromyography, serve as excellent biomarkers for diagnosis but do not adequately substitute for clinical evaluations to predict treatment response. New technologies are emerging that enable broad biomarker discovery in biological fluids. Biomarker evaluation is ideally done in the context of longitudinal clinical trials. The MGTX trial has collected plasma and serum for RNA and protein analysis and thymus, which will allow robust biomarker discovery. The ultimate goal will be to identify candidates for a reliable substitute for a clinically meaningful end point that is a direct measure of the effectiveness of a therapy in the context of a continuum of disease natural history and a patient's overall well-being.

Keywords: biomarkers; myasthenia gravis; surrogate end point; Prentice criteria

The Food and Drug Administration (FDA), National Institutes of Health (NIH), and the pharmaceutical/device maker industry have placed a major focus on the identification of biomarkers to assist therapeutic development in preclinical and early phase studies on humans.[1,2] Why? Despite some remarkable success in discovery of novel treatments, therapeutic development has a high failure rate.[3–5] Numerous forces are now driving limitations on financial support for discovery of new treatments, whether scientists work in the private or public sector. Biomarkers in animal studies, which support efficacy in humans and ones that can robustly support go/no-go decisions in preliminary clinical trials, offer promise to decrease the failure rate, shorten the duration, and thereby reduce the cost of therapeutic development.

Biomarker categorization

The U.S. FDA defines biomarkers as characteristics that are objectively measured and evaluated as indicators of normal biologic processes, pathogenic activity, or pharmacologic responses to a therapeutic intervention.[6] Biomarkers may be assessed by a variety of measures from biological specimens, such as molecular genetic characteristics, histology, and serum proteins as well as imaging evaluations. Several varieties of biomarkers exist (Table 1). For example, prognostic biomarkers sort patients according to the likely course of disease (if left untreated), while predictive biomarkers identify subpopulations of patients who are likely to respond to a specific therapy. The drug dosage for responsive individuals is optimized by analysis of pharmacodynamic biomarkers. Biomarkers may predict or identify safety problems related to a therapeutic candidate. In some circumstances, a biomarker may identify a patient population subgroup that becomes the focus for specific clinical trials. These include prognostic biomarkers that identify patients with a disease risk most suitable for an efficient drug development program. In other circumstances, a

doi: 10.1111/j.1749-6632.2012.06787.x

Table 1. Categorization of biomarkers

Biomarker	Example	Disease
Diagnostic	Elevated fasting blood sugar	Diabetes mellitus
	Acetylcholine receptor and muscle-specific antibody	Myasthenia gravis
Disease extent/severity	Lesion burden on magnetic resonance imaging	Multiple sclerosis
	Tumor size	Various neoplasms
Pharmacodynamic marker	Serum cyclooxygenase (COX)-2 inhibition	Pain relief
Prognostic marker	Estrogen receptor status	Breast cancer
Predictive marker	Serum cholesterol	Cardio- and cerebrovascular disease
	Blood pressure	
Drug characterization	Complement inhibition (by drug eculizumab)	Paroxysmal hemoglobinuria

predictive biomarker may identify a patient subgroup that has a greater potential to benefit from the mechanism of action of the specific drug or a lower risk of an identified adverse effect of the drug. As with any measure, there are variability and specificity issues that must be considered for each specific application. The rigor of the validation process for a biomarker is dependent on its ultimate clinical use.

The surrogate end point is of greatest interest for therapeutic development, and their validation as a predictor of efficacy requires fulfillment of strict criteria. The surrogate end point is intended to substitute for a primary clinical end point and is expected to predict a clinical benefit, lack of benefit, or harm as would the gold standard clinical end point. Prentice originally proposed criteria to define expectations for a surrogate (Table 2). To act as a surrogate end point a biomarker must fulfill these properties, which are ideally assessed in the context of a clinical trial.[7] Of course, this also assumes that clinical efficacy evaluations have been validated appropriately, which is also a challenge. Only in the case of death as a clinical end point can one consider the clinical measures to be unequivocal.

Biomarkers in myasthenia gravis

The MG research field lags behind other areas of medicine in the development of biomarkers, and existing biomarkers are severely limited in their ability to predict a response to treatment, assess susceptibility to adverse effects of treatment, or correlate with disease severity. This lack of validated biomarkers is a glaring deficiency for therapeutic development for MG, especially when novel treatments are being considered for application. This state is all the more surprising because MG is one of the best characterized autoimmune disorders from a biological perspective and is among the few that fulfills strict criteria for autoimmunity.

Biomarkers that presently exist in MG fall primarily in the diagnostic category. Detection of acetylcholine receptor (AChR) or muscle-specific kinase (MuSK) antibodies is highly specific for confirming the diagnosis of MG; however, their absolute levels do not correlate with disease severity.[8–10] Although levels of AChR and MuSK antibodies tend to fall with treatment, this is highly variable and does not correlate well with disease severity or clinical response. The therapeutic usefulness of biomarkers in guiding treatment decisions is illustrated by the identification of MuSK antibodies, which correlate with poor response to cholinesterase inhibitor treatment and often predict refractoriness to other treatment approaches. However, such observations have been drawn from retrospective analyses.

The Myasthenia Gravis Foundation of America Task Force for evaluation of clinical end points, of which three of the authors (H.K., G.W., G.C.) were members, reviewed potential biomarkers used in MG. None fulfills criteria sufficiently to serve as surrogate end points. Acetylcholine receptor (AChR) antibody titers have been used as a marker for therapeutic response,[11–13] but there is no basis to use them as a potential substitute for a clinical outcome measure. Single-fiber EMG, in expert hands, appears to correlate well to clinical state; however, it is of limited use as a predictor of clinical outcome, especially owing to the likelihood of significant

Table 2. Prentice criteria for surrogate end point validation

Treatment must have an effect on the surrogate

Treatment must have an effect on the clinical outcome

Surrogate and the clinical outcome must be correlated

Treatment effect on the true clinical outcome must disappear when adjusting for the surrogate

interobserver variability.[14] Of relevance to MG treatment is the thiopurine *S*-methyltransferase activity or identification of the TPMT gene mutation as a marker of toxicity for azathioprine use.[15]

Genetic markers may one day serve as biomarkers important for therapeutic targeting. A genetic association for MG is supported[16] by (1) MG occurrence in up to 4% of family members of patients with MG, while the risk of generalized MG in the population is 0.01%; (2) twin studies showing a heritability index of 0.65, a level that places MG in the range of Alzheimer's disease and epilepsy and above multiple sclerosis for genetic predisposition; (3) HLA-B8 and DR3 alleles are increased in patients with MG when compared with the general population; (4) the MYSA1 locus is associated with MG and thymic hyperplasia; MYSA1 lies within the central region of the HLA region and the biological basis for it leading to susceptibility to MG has not been determined; (5) linkage dysequilibrium analysis identified an association with a marker in the CHRNA1 gene, which codes for the alpha subunit of the ACHR, that has been closely associated with MG; and (6) a polymorphism identified in the promoter region of the decay accelerating factor (DAF) gene, a complement regulator associated with a severe form of MG that produces irreversible ophthalmoparesis.[17]

Preclinical evaluation

Development of therapeutics is dependent on exploratory evaluations in animals, and the field of MG benefits greatly from the existence of robust animal models. Patrick and Lindstrom demonstrated that immunization of rabbits with purified acetylcholine receptor leads to development of disease that mimics the human disorder.[18] Subsequent studies have demonstrated that experimental autoimmune

MG (EAMG) can be induced in several mammalian species by immunization with AChR of mammals, the electric organ of eels or rays, and peptide fragments of AChR subunits.[19] These models reproduce aspects of human MG, including a breakdown in tolerance with production of autoantibodies, the neuromuscular transmission defect, response to anticholinesterase therapy, and moderation of the disease by treatments used in patients. EAMG produced by administration of antibodies to the acetylcholine receptor fails to mimic the breakdown in tolerance and induces significant inflammation, which is not present in muscles of the patient, but does mimic the final common pathway of injury to the neuromuscular junction that occurs in humans, and therefore, also serves as an appropriate model to evaluate certain therapeutics. These models have been used to delineate autoimmune mechanisms and to evaluate therapeutics[20,21] but to date have not been a focus for biomarker discovery.

Because of inherent differences between humans and animals, no animal model, thus far, fully mimics the human disease. Despite common features of mammalian immune systems, there are differences in basic regulatory proteins of human, mouse, and rat systems. EAMG differs from human MG in the need to administer exogenous and repeated antigenic stimulation to produce and maintain disease. Fluctuations of weakness and autoimmune activity are not observed over time. Therefore, caution is necessary when extrapolating positive results from animals to humans. This is not just a problem for MG. A glaring example is over 300 preclinical studies of Alzheimer's disease suggesting efficacy of therapy in mouse models, none of which have led to a therapeutic effect in humans.[22] Therefore, there is a great need for biomarker discovery to be integrated coherently into both preclinical and clinical efforts. The long-term benefit that would result from validated markers of efficacy in humans would be enormous. And if these discoveries have parallels in animal studies the potential to translate novel treatments from preclinical studies to the bedside would be far more efficient. Of course, there is also benefit in the early termination of preclinical efforts that have little chance for success in order to save the hundreds of millions of dollars that are expended on human early phase trials.

MGTX study and biomarker discovery opportunity

In 2005 the NIH funded a multicenter, international, single-blinded, randomized trial (MGTX) to determine whether extended transsternal thymectomy for patients receiving the prednisone protocol confers added benefits to the prednisone protocol alone.[23,24] As part of the investigation, an ancillary study was supported with the intent to collect thymus, plasma, serum and blood-derived RNA with the intent of developing the first biomarker discovery assessment in the history of MG. As of this writing, 82 subjects have provided blood specimens at baseline and six-month follow-up with collection ongoing at one, two, and three years postrandomization. Over 50 thymic specimens have been collected, and analysis for histological evaluation has demonstrated good-to-excellent quality of specimen integrity. The opportunity exists now to launch a state-of-the-art, unbiased biomarker discovery program utilizing these specimens. To that end, the authors are moving toward the use of independent-omics assays (proteomics, microRNA, RNA profiling, metabolomics) coupled with antigen-specific IgG subclass definition on samples obtained through MGTX and to perform similar analyses on samples obtained from mice with EAMG. Below we briefly describe the methods to be used.

Nanoparticle proteomics

Body fluids, such as serum, are valuable sources of biomarker information. Identification and monitoring of circulating biomarkers enable early disease detection, disease/morbidity risk stratification, and help assess disease progression and thus responsiveness to interventions.[25] Despite recent progress in the field of proteomics, identification of novel plasma biomarkers such as proteins has been difficult due to low quantities relative to larger and more abundant plasma proteins, such as albumin.[26] Nanoparticle proteomic technology will allow identification and quantitation of less abundant proteins within patient samples.

MicroRNA profiling

MicroRNA (miRNA) has emerged as a new and important class of cellular regulators. Experimental studies have provided strong evidence that aberrant expression of miRNA is associated with a broad spectrum of human diseases, including cancer, diabetes, and cardiovascular and psychological disorders. The relatively small numbers of miRNAs discovered in humans ($\sim$800 miRNAs, miRBase12.0) are involved in regulation of a large number of human genes (up to 80% of known genes). miRNAs have exceptional potential as biomarkers because of their relative abundance, highly specific expression, and stable presence in serum and plasma. In fact, circulating miRNAs demonstrate reasonable sensitivity in a small number of Duchenne muscular dystrophy patients as biomarkers for disease progression and severity and also correlate with circulating miRNA in mice with dystrophin deficiency.[27]

Metabolomics profiling

Metabolomics is a rapidly developing field that aims to identify and quantify the concentration changes of all the metabolites (i.e., the metabolome) in a given biofluid from a subject and support targeting and developing therapeutics.[28] The anticipated contribution of metabolomics to the field of science and to healthcare is highlighted by its presence in the current NIH Roadmap. The application of metabolomics to understand the manifestation and progression of complex neurological diseases is a powerful means of identifying the earliest markers associated with disease progression and treatment response.

MG-focused assessments

The final effector mechanism in most patients with MG is the AChR antibody.[29] A fundamental challenge for the MG field is that the level of the autoantibody does not correlate with disease severity. Numerous investigations have demonstrated that there is a significant role of complement as a driver of disease pathology in experimental animals and humans with MG. In concert with the broad-based assessments, we will specifically evaluate IgG subclasses, that are specific to the human AChR autoantigen. It is also well appreciated that cytokines regulate the cell responses of the immune system; multiplex cytometric bead assays can be used to measure levels of serum cytokines[30] to determine the treatment effect on these biomarkers, although these may be too volatile to be used as effective biomarkers.

Identification is not enough

Identifying putative biomarkers is a major endeavor in all diseases in the era of personalized medicine, but the challenge in establishing a biomarker should not be underestimated. The Prentice criteria are theoretical and have not been achieved even where biomarkers are felt to exist (e.g., blood pressure for cardiovascular disease or CD4[+] T cell counts for HIV). Although the path to validation of a biomarker is long and arduous, the payoff is enormous for patients, the field of research, and is now a reasonable undertaking with the tools that are at hand.

Conclusion

The time has come for further breakthroughs in treatment of MG. The only path forward lies in exploiting approaches that the field of cancer therapeutics is beginning to leverage. These include rigorously evaluated clinical end points and identification of biomarkers for subcategorization of neoplasms on a molecular level indicative of potential therapeutic targets in clinical trials. One such success story is that of chronic myelogenous leukemia, which began with discovery of the Philadelphia chromosome and finally led to the targeting of an antibody to inhibit a tyrosine kinase.[31] The drug developed is Gleevec, a highly effective treatment for this subset of leukemia patients. MG faces particular challenges in that universally accepted clinical end points have only recently been rigorously defined[32,33] and research consortiums to perform robust clinical trials are only a decade old. The field also faces the challenge of a lack of investigators trained in biomarker discovery. However, it is expected that the MGTX-supported biological specimen bank will offer many investigators a unique opportunity to move the field forward for the benefit of generations of patients to come.

Acknowledgments

This work was supported by NINDS Grant U01 NS042685.

Conflicts of interest

The authors declare no conflicts of interest.

References

1. Butterfield, L.H., A.K. Palucka, C.M. Britten, *et al.* 2011. Recommendations from the iSBTc-SITC/FDA/NCI workshop on immunotherapy biomarkers. *Clin. Cancer Res.* **17:** 3064–3076.

2. http://www.biomarkersconsortium.org. Accessed Sept 4, 2012.

3. Mendell, J.R., C. Csimma, C.M. McDonald, *et al.* 2007. Challenges in drug development for muscle disease: a stakeholders' meeting. *Muscle Nerve* **35:** 8–16.

4. Kola, I. 2008. The state of innovation in drug development. *Clin. Pharmacol. Therap.* **83:** 227–231.

5. Paul, S.M., D.S. Mytelka, C.T. Dunwiddie, *et al.* 2010. How to improve R&D productivity: the pharmaceutical industry's grand challenge. *Nat. Rev. Drug Discov.* **9:** 203–214.

6. US Food and Drug Administration. Available at: http://www.fda.gov/ScienceResearch/SpecialTopics/CriticalPath Initiative/ucm076689.htm. Accessed September 4, 2012.

7. Prentice, R.L. 1989. Surrogate endpoints in clinical trials: definition and operational criteria. *Stat. Med.* **8:** 431–440.

8. Howard, F.J., V. Lennon, J. Finley, *et al.* 1987. Clinical correlations of antibodies that bind, block, or modulate human acetylcholine receptors in myasthenia gravis. *Ann. N.Y. Acad. Sci.* **505:** 526–538.

9. Lennon, V. 1997. Serologic profile of myasthenia gravis and distinction from Lambert-Eaton myasthenic syndrome. *Neurology* **48** (**Suppl 5**): S23–S27.

10. Guptill, J.T. & D.B. Sanders. 2010. Update on muscle-specific tyrosine kinase antibody positive myasthenia gravis. *Curr. Opin. Neurol.* **23:** 530–535.

11. Palace, J., J. Newsom-Davis & B Lecky. 1998. A randomized double-blind trial of prednisolone alone or with azathioprine in myasthenia gravis. Myasthenia Gravis Study Group. *Neurology* **50:** 1778–1783.

12. Muscle Study, G. 2008. A trial of mycophenolate mofetil with prednisone as initial immunotherapy in myasthenia gravis. *Neurology* **71:** 394–399.

13. Sanders, D.B., I.K. Hart, R. Mantegazza, *et al.* 2008. An international, phase III, randomized trial of mycophenolate mofetil in myasthenia gravis. *Neurology* **71:** 400–406.

14. Sanders, D.B. 2004. Electrophysiologic tests of neuromuscular transmission. *Suppl. Clin. Neurophysiol.* **57:** 167–169.

15. Colleoni, L., D. Kapetis, L. Maggi, *et al.* 2012. A new thiopurine S-methyltransferase haplotype associated with intolerance to azathioprine. *J. Clin. Pharmacol.* Feb 3. [Epub ahead of print].

16. Lanford, J.W. & L.H. Phillips. 2009. Epidemiology and Genetics of Myasthenia Gravis. H.J. Kaminski, Ed.: 71–78. New York. Springer.

17. Heckmann, J.M., H. Uwimpuhwe, R. Ballo, *et al.* 2010. A functional SNP in the regulatory region of the decay-accelerating factor gene associates with extraocular muscle pareses in myasthenia gravis. *Genes Immun.* **11:** 1–10.

18. Patrick, J. & J. Lindstrom. 1973. Autoimmune response to acetylcholine receptor. *Science* **180:** 871–872.

19. Christadoss P, M. Poussin & C. Deng. 2000. Animal models of myasthenia gravis. *Clin. Immunol.* **94:** 75–87.

20. Vincent, A. 2010. Autoimmune channelopathies: well-established and emerging immunotherapy-responsive diseases of the peripheral and central nervous systems. *J. Clin. Immunol.* **30**(Suppl 1): S97–S102.

21. Conti-Fine, B.M., M. Milani & H.J. Kaminski. 2006. Myasthenia gravis: past, present, and future. *J. Clin. Invest.* **116:** 2843–2854.

22. Shineman, D.W., G.S. Basi, J.L. Bizon, *et al.* 2011. Accelerating drug discovery for Alzheimer's disease: best practices for preclinical animal studies. *Alzheimer's Res. Ther.* **3:** 28.

23. Minisman, G., M. Bhanushali, R. Conwit, *et al.* 2012. Implementing clinical trials on an international platform: challenges and perspectives. *J. Neurol. Sci.* **313:** 1–6.

24. Newsom-Davis, J., G. Cutter, G.I. Wolfe, *et al.* 2008. Status of the thymectomy trial for nonthymomatous myasthenia gravis patients receiving prednisone. *Ann. N.Y. Acad. Sci.* **1132:** 344–347.

25. Hanash, S. 2003. Disease proteomics. *Nature* **422:** 226–232.

26. Longo C, A. Patanarut, T. George, *et al.* 2009. Core-shell hydrogel particles harvest, concentrate and preserve labile low abundance biomarkers. *PLoS One* **4:** e4763.

27. Cacchiarelli D, I. Legnini, J. Martone, *et al.* 2011. miRNAs as serum biomarkers for Duchenne muscular dystrophy. *EMBO Mol. Med.* **3:** 258–265.

28. Kaddurah-Daouk, R., B.S. Kristal & R.M. Weinshilboum. 2008. Metabolomics: a global biochemical approach to drug response and disease. *Annu. Rev. Pharmacol. Toxicol.* **48:** 653–683.

29. Kusner, L.L., H.J. Kaminski & J. Soltys. 2008. Effect of complement and its regulation on myasthenia gravis pathogenesis. *Expert Rev. Clin. Immunol.* **4:** 43–52.

30. Tuzun, E., R. Huda & P. Christadoss. 2011. Complement and cytokine based therapeutic strategies in myasthenia gravis. *J. Autoimmun.* **37:** 136–143.

31. Capdeville, R., E. Buchdunger, J. Zimmermann, *et al.* 2002. Glivec (STI571, imatinib), a rationally developed, targeted anticancer drug. *Nat. Rev. Drug Discov.* **1:** 493–502.

32. Benatar, M., D.B. Sanders, T.M. Burns, *et al.* 2012. Recommendations for myasthenia gravis clinical trials. *Muscle Nerve* **45:** 909–917.

33. Jaretzki, A., 3rd, R.J. Barohn, R.M. Ernstoff, *et al.* 2000. Myasthenia gravis: recommendations for clinical research standards. Task Force of the Medical Scientific Advisory Board of the Myasthenia Gravis Foundation of America. *Neurology* **55:** 16–23.

Ann. N.Y. Acad. Sci. ISSN 0077-8923

Experimental myasthenia gravis in Aire-deficient mice: a link between Aire and regulatory T cells

Revital Aricha,[1] Tali Feferman,[1] Sonia Berrih-Aknin,[2] Sara Fuchs,[1] and Miriam C. Souroujon[1,3]

[1]Department of Immunology, The Weizmann Institute of Science, Rehovot, Israel. [2]INSERM U996, France. [3]Department of Natural Sciences, The Open University of Israel, Raanana, Israel

Address for correspondence: Sara Fuchs, Department of Immunology, The Weizmann Institute of Science, Rehovot, Israel 76100. sara.fuchs@weizmann.ac.il

Aire (autoimmune regulator) has a key role in the establishment of tolerance to autoantigens. Aire$^{-/-}$ mice present decreased thymic expression of AChR, significantly lower frequencies of regulatory T (T_{reg}) cells, and higher expression of Th17 markers, compared to controls. We therefore predicted that Aire$^{-/-}$ mice would be more susceptible to induction of experimental autoimmune myasthenia gravis (EAMG). However, when EAMG was induced in young mice, Aire$^{-/-}$ mice presented a milder disease that wild-type (WT) controls. In contrast, when EAMG was induced in older mice, Aire$^{-/-}$ mice were more severely affected than WT mice. The relative resistance to EAMG in young Aire$^{-/-}$ mice correlated with increased numbers of T_{reg} cells in their spleens compared to young controls. A similar age-related susceptibility was also observed when EAE was induced in Aire$^{-/-}$ mice, suggesting an age-related link among Aire, disease susceptibility, and peripheral T_{reg} cells that may be a general feature of autoimmunity.

Keywords: Aire; regulatory T cells; experimental autoimmune myasthenia gravis (EAMG); thymus; spleen

Central tolerance and Aire

Thymic tolerance plays an important role in preventing autoimmunity. At an immature stage of development, autoreactive T cell precursors are exposed to self-antigens within the thymus and as a result undergo negative selection. The establishment of thymic tolerance occurs mainly in the medullary compartment of the thymus.[1] Medullary thymic epithelial cells (mTECs) ectopically express a large array of gene products, including tissue-restricted antigens (TRAs) that are normally present only in specialized peripheral organs and are apparently not required for the direct function of mTECs. Despite the substantial impact of central thymic tolerance to self-antigens, some autoreactive T cells leave the thymus. Such cells are kept under control by peripheral tolerance mechanisms that include suppressive activity of regulatory T (T_{reg}) cells. T_{reg} cell abnormalities have been reported in several autoimmune diseases in humans and in their respective experimental models. The thymic expression of many of the TRAs is dependent on the autoimmune regulator (Aire) gene product, a transcription factor that is highly expressed in medullary thymic epithe-

lial cells (mTECs).[2] Aire promotes the ectopic expression of the peripheral TRAs in mTECs, thereby leading to tolerance toward self-antigens. Mutation of Aire in patients is solely responsible for the development of autoimmune-polyendocrinopathy-candidiasis ectodermal dystrophy (APECED), a rare autoimmune disease. Aire deficiency leads to lymphoid cell infiltrates associated with deposition of autoantibodies and severe, multiorgan, tissue-specific autoimmunity in a variety of peripheral tissues of both mice and humans,[2–7] thus reinforcing the importance of Aire's role in controlling immune tolerance.[1] T_{reg} cells were shown to be impaired in APECED patients, suggesting that a T_{reg} cell defect is involved in the pathogenesis of disease. This was manifested by a significantly decreased expression of Foxp3 mRNA and protein and decreased T_{reg} cell function.[6]

Autoimmune myasthenia gravis: T_{reg} cells and Aire

T_{reg} cells play a critical role in the immunopathogenesis of myasthenia gravis. Thymic T_{reg} cells were shown to be functionally impaired in MG patients,[8]

doi: 10.1111/j.1749-6632.2012.06843.x

and the frequency of $CD4^+$ $CD25^+$ T_{reg} cells in peripheral lymphocytes of MG patients seems to be lower than that of healthy subjects.[9] Following successful immunsuppression or thymectomy, $CD4^+$ $CD25^{high}$ cells of MG patients reach normal or elevated numbers, compared to healthy controls.[10,11] Several groups have evaluated peripheral blood cells from MG patients to determine T_{reg} cell number and function. These studies have shown a normal to decreased population of $CD4^+CD25^{high}$ cells in peripheral blood of MG patients compared to healthy controls.[10,12,13] We have previously observed in experimental autoimmune MG (EAMG) in rats, that at early stages of disease, the frequency of $CD4^+$ $CD25^{high}$ $Foxp3^+$ cells is lower in PBL of myasthenic rats compared to healthy controls. Moreover, we have shown that administration of T_{reg} cells that were generated *ex vivo*, from healthy rats to myasthenic rats suppressed EAMG and led to downregulation of humoral AChR-specific responses.[14]

A possible involvement of Aire in the development of MG was suggested by the finding that mTEC isolated from Aire-deficient mice contain significant lower levels of mRNA transcripts for CHRNA 1, a gene coding for AChR, compared to wild-type (WT) mTECs.[15] In addition, Giraud *et al.*[16] have shown that AChR expression levels in human thymus has an impact on MG development since disease onset in EOMG patients with lower AChR expression levels was earlier. However, the absence of Aire expression in thymomas was per se not associated with MG and is commonly insufficient to elicit APECED or even features of APECED,[17] with rare exceptions.[18]

We have observed that Aire mRNA expression in the thymus is correlated with susceptibility to EAMG in different mouse strains.[19] C57BL/6 mice, which are susceptible to the induction of EAMG, have significantly lower thymic mRNA expression levels of Aire, compared to SJL and Balb/c mice that are resistant to EAMG induction. In addition, the mRNA expression of the AChR α- and β-subunits is lower in the thymus of the EAMG-susceptible C57BL/6 mice compared with the EAMG-resistant SJL and Balb/c mice (Fig. 1A). Moreover, thymic expression of the AChR α-subunit in Aire knockout (KO) mice is significantly lower than in WT mice (Fig. 1B).[19]

Susceptibility of Aire$^{-/-}$ mice to EAMG is age related

The phenotype of Aire deficiency in mice has been characterized by a limited number of spontaneous autoimmune diseases. Even though AChR is one of the TSA genes that are controlled by Aire, the involvement of Aire in the pathogenesis of EAMG has not been demonstrated. In a recent study[19] we found that Aire knockout (KO) mice express lower levels of the AChR α-subunit in their thymus compared to WT mice, as was also reported before.[15] However, the expression of the AChR β-subunit was similar to its expression in WT mice. It should be noted that although the α-subunit is the most immunogenic subunit in AChR and is the target of the majority of the anti-AChR autoantibody response, the lack of effect of the Aire deficiency on the expression of AChR subunits and the partial effect on the AChR α-subunit might explain why MG is not a feature of APECED patients and why EAMG does not appear spontaneously in Aire KO mice. However, the loss of central tolerance to TRAs might render Aire KO mice to be more susceptible to the induction of EAMG, as has been recently shown for another experimentally induced autoimmune disease namely collagen-induced arthritis.[20]

By analyzing the role of the Aire gene in the susceptibility of mice to EAMG we have observed an increased susceptibility to EAMG in Aire KO mice that was evident only in older mice (i.e., not in young mice under five months of age). This age-related susceptibility was shown to be associated with changes in T_{reg} cells.[19] When two-month-old Aire KO mice (the optimal age for EAMG induction in mice) and WT mice were immunized with Torpedo AChR, unexpectedly, the KO mice had milder EAMG (mean clinical score 0.38) until approximately 10 weeks following immunization, compared with the WT group (mean clinical score 1.05). However, three months after immunization, when the mice were about five months old, this pattern changed and the Aire KO mice presented higher clinical scores compared to WT mice (mean clinical score at the end of the experiment: 1.88 and 0.88 for the Aire KO and WT groups, respectively (Fig. 2). In order to find out whether the susceptibility of Aire KO mice to EAMG is higher, compared to WT controls, only in older mice, EAMG was induced in six-month-old mice, the same age in which EAMG was more

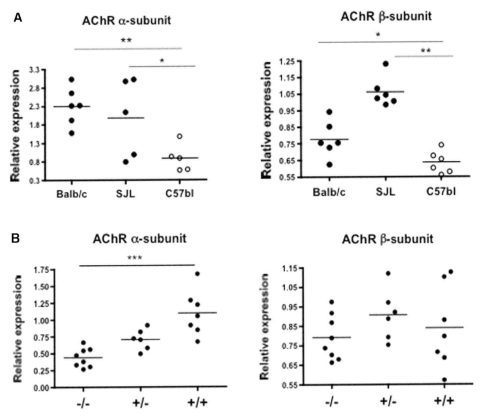

Figure 1. AChR mRNA expression levels. Thymuses from different mouse strains (Balb/c, SJL, and C57BL/6) (A) or of Aire$^{-/-}$, heterozygotes$^{+/-}$, and WT$^{+/+}$ mice (B) were obtained from eight-week-old mice, and mRNA expression levels were analyzed by quantitative real time RT-PCR. GAPDH was used as an inner control for normalization for each cytokine. Error bars indicate SEM values ($n = 6$) $^{*}P < 0.05$; $^{**}P < 0.005$; $^{***}P < 0.0005$. Data are from Ref. 19.

severe in the Aire KO mice immunized at the age of two months. Indeed, when EAMG was induced in six-month-old mice, the Aire KO mice presented a more severe disease than the WT mice throughout the experiment. At 12 weeks following EAMG induction the mean clinical scores were 1.83 and 0.81 for the Aire KO and WT groups, respectively.

Is there a link between Aire and T$_{reg}$ cells?

There is a clear synergy between mutations in Foxp3 and Aire, since the disease in double-deficient animals was accelerated compared to either of the single mutants.[2] However, the link between Aire and T$_{reg}$ cells is still not fully resolved (Ref. 3 and references therein). Several previous studies have reported that Aire does not seem to influence the T$_{reg}$ cell compartment at a global level.[5–7,21] However, some recent studies suggest that Aire-expressing mTECs are involved in the generation of TRA-specific Foxp3^{+}

T$_{reg}$ cells. Aschenbrenner *et al.*[22] have shown that Aire^{+} mTECs expressing TRAs facilitate the development of TRA-specific T$_{reg}$ cells in the thymus and suggested that a small number of TRA-specific T$_{reg}$ cells may contribute to the occurrence of autoimmune diseases in Aire-deficient mice and human APECED patients. A recent study by Hinterberger *et al.*[23] supports this concept by showing that Aire-expressing mTECs, in addition to providing an antigen reservoir, also serve as antigen-presenting cells, thus enhancing the selection of T$_{reg}$ cells. The commitment of the T$_{reg}$ cell lineage was shown to occur independently of Foxp3, and interaction of developing thymocytes with thymic stromal cells may drive the differentiation of a thymocyte subpopulation into the T$_{reg}$ cell lineage and subsequently trigger the expression of Foxp3.[24] Lymphocytes from patients with the APECED syndrome were evaluated by quantitative real-time PCR and by flow

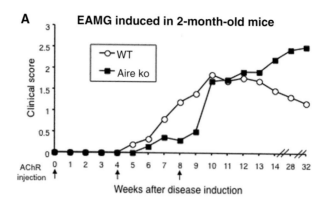

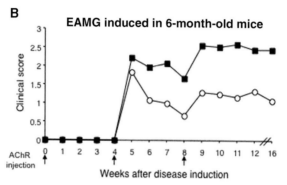

Figure 2. Susceptibility of Aire KO mice to EAMG. Aire KO and WT mice ($n = 12$ per group) were immunized by Torpedo AChR in CFA at the age of two months (A) or at the age of six months (B) and boosted twice at four-week intervals. Arrows indicate the time points of AChR immunizations. Mice were scored twice weekly for clinical signs of EAMG on a scale of 0–4, as previously described.[14] Data represent one out of three independent experiments. $P < 0.05$ for (A) and $P < 0.0005$ in (B), analyzed by the two-way ANOVA test and the paired nonparametric (Wilcoxon) test. Data from Ref. 19.

cytometry to address the possibility that Aire plays a role in the generation of functional T_{reg} cells. Consistently, the percentage of $CD4^+$ $CD25^{high}$ cells in these patients was decreased, the amount of Foxp3 expressed per cell was reduced, and the capability to suppress effector T cells was diminished.[6,25] More recently, Laakso *et al.*[26] demonstrated that APECED patients have T_{reg} cell abnormalities associated with loss of naive Foxp3+ precursors and suggested that autoimmunity in these Aire-deficient patients is associated with a deregulated peripheral T_{reg} cell homeostasis.

Our recent study in EAMG rats may shed some light on the link between Aire and T_{reg} cells. We have observed a significant ($P = 0.0004$) and reproducible reduction (22%) in the proportion of $CD4^+$ Foxp3+ T cells in the thymus of Aire KO mice compared to WT controls.[19] This is in contrast to earlier studies concluding that there are no significant abnormalities in T_{reg} cells of Aire KO mice.[5,7,21]

However, a closer look at some of these reports reveals a trend of reduction in the proportion of $CD4^+$ Foxp3+ T_{reg} cells in the Aire KO mice, as was also discussed by Hubert *et al.*[5] The large sample size we have used in our studies has enabled us to detect a highly significant and reproducible reduction in the proportion of $CD4^+$ Foxp3+ T cells in the thymus of Aire KO mice compared to WT controls that may have not been revealed in other studies. In addition, although others and we have used Aire KO mice on a C57BL background, we cannot rule out the possibility that the statistical differences between the results reflect subtle differences between the source of Aire KO mouse strains and their extent of Aire loss.

We found in the periphery a higher percentage of $CD4^+$ Foxp3+ cells in the spleens of two-month-old Aire KO mice (Fig. 3A) that correlated with their relative resistance to EAMG at this time point. However, in older (six-month-old) mice, the Aire

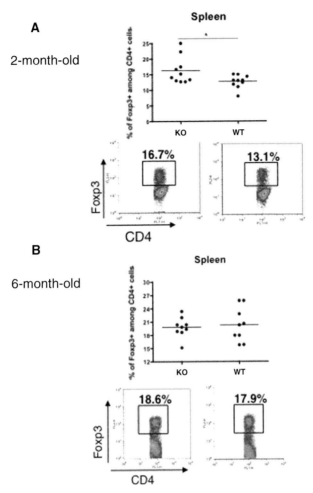

Figure 3. T$_{reg}$ cell numbers in the spleen of Aire KO and WT mice. FACS analysis of CD4$^+$ Foxp3$^+$ in two-month-old mice (A) and six-month-old mice (B). Horizontal bars in A and B top panels indicate mean values ($n = 10$). Four independent experiments were performed. Representative FACS profiles of individual mice of the indicated genotype are shown in A and B bottom panels. $^*P < 0.05$; $^{***}P < 0.0005$. Data are from Ref. 19.

KO mice lost their relative resistance to disease, concomitant to the reduced proportion of T$_{reg}$ cell in the periphery of naive Aire KO mice (Fig. 3B). The higher CD4$^+$ Foxp3$^+$ cell content in the spleen of two-month-old Aire KO mice could result from either an enhanced export of CD4$^+$ Foxp3$^+$ cells from the thymus to the spleen or alternatively, by their increased proliferation within the spleen. The first possibility has been ruled out, since there was no increase in the number of naive CD4$^+$ Foxp3$^+$ CD62L$^+$ cells in the spleen of Aire KO mice (Fig. 4, right panel) compared to controls. This result indicates that there is no defect in the thymic output of naive CD4$^+$ Foxp3$^-$ CD62L$^+$ cells to the periphery in Aire KO mice, meaning that the lower number of naive T$_{reg}$ cells in the periphery of Aire KO mice do not stem from reduced numbers of CD4$^+$ Foxp3$^+$ cells migrating from their thymus. The second alternative, namely, that the increased number of T$_{reg}$ cells in the spleen of two-month-old Aire KO mice result from their increased proliferation within the spleen proved to be the right one. Indeed, a higher proportion of Ki67-expressing CD4$^+$ Foxp3$^+$ cells was observed in the spleen of Aire KO mice compared to WT controls (Fig. 4, left panel). This observation is supported by a study reporting that APECED patients have an increased expression of Ki67 in their peripheral T$_{reg}$ cells.[26] Moreover, a

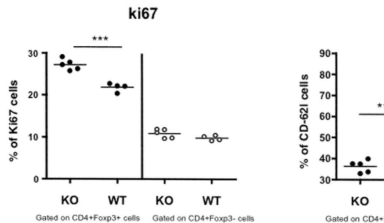
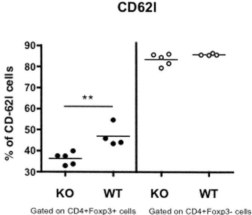

Figure 4. Ki67 and CD62l expression in CD4$^+$ Foxp3 splenocytes of Aire KO and WT mice. FACS analysis of the percent of Ki67$^+$ and CD62L$^+$ cells within CD4$^+$ Foxp3$^+$ (black circles) and CD4$^+$ Foxp3$^-$ (open circles) cells in the spleen of two-month-old mice. Horizontal bars indicate mean values ($n = 5$). $^{**}P < 0.005$; $^{***}P < 0.0005$. Data are from Ref. 19.

decreased thymic output was shown to induce compensatory auto proliferation of peripheral T cells.[27]

We wondered whether the increased proportion of peripheral T_{reg} cells in two-month-old Aire KO mice and the reduction in the proportion of peripheral T_{reg} cells with age is specific to EAMG, or whether it is a more general phenomenon that may be seen also in other models of autoimmune diseases. For that we have tested the susceptibility of mice to experimental autoimmune encephalomyelitis (EAE) induced by myelin oligonucleotide glycoprotein (MOG) in Aire KO mice compared to WT controls. Indeed, we have preliminary data (in collaboration with Rina Aharoni) indicating that the susceptibility of Aire KO mice to MOG-induced EAE increases as they age and is also correlated with the state of T_{reg} cells in the periphery. These observations may suggest that the age-related changes in susceptibility of Aire KO mice to autoimmune disease induction and their link to the state of peripheral T_{reg} cells are not restricted to EAMG and may be a more general feature of autoimmune diseases.

Summary

Our results suggest that Aire expression is involved in the induction of EAMG. However, additional factors seem to be required for the expression of a fully developed disease in Aire KO mice. Aire KO mice have reduced T_{reg} cell numbers in their thymus, and the induction and course of EAMG in these mice is

age dependent and correlates with changes in T_{reg} cell numbers in the periphery. It is therefore reasonable to assume that an alteration in the T_{reg} cell compartment is one of the factors that facilitate the development of autoreactive T cells, thereby leading to the development of EAMG. Taken together, this study points to a putative link between Aire and Foxp3-expressing regulatory T cells and suggests a role for both in the susceptibility to, and pathogenesis of, myasthenia gravis and possibly other autoimmune diseases.

Acknowledgments

The work described in this paper was supported by grants from the Muscular Dystrophy Association of America (MDA), the Association Francaise Contre les Myopathies (AFM), the European Commission (FIGHT-MG, contract # FP7 HEALTH-2009-242-210), and the Open University of Israel Research Fund.

Conflicts of interest

The authors declare no conflicts of interest.

References

1. Peterson, P., T. Org & A. Rebane. 2008. Transcriptional regulation by AIRE: molecular mechanisms of central tolerance. *Nat. Rev Immunol.* **8:** 948–957.
2. Anderson, M.S., *et al.* 2005. The cellular mechanism of Aire control of T cell tolerance. *Immunity* **23:** 227–239.
3. Nomura, T. & S. Sakaguchi. 2007. Foxp3 and Aire in thymus-generated Treg cells: a link in self-tolerance. *Nat. Immunol.* **8:** 333–334.

4. Gardner, J. M. *et al.* 2008. Deletional tolerance mediated by extrathymic Aire-expressing cells. *Science* **321**: 843–847.

5. Hubert, F. X. *et al.* 2009. Aire-deficient C57BL/6 mice mimicking the common human 13-base pair deletion mutation present with only a mild autoimmune phenotype. *J. Immunol.* **182**: 3902–3918.

6. Kekalainen, E. *et al.* 2007. A defect of regulatory T cells in patients with autoimmune polyendocrinopathy-candidiasis-ectodermal dystrophy. *J. Immunol.* **178**: 1208–1215.

7. Kuroda, N. *et al.* 2005. Development of autoimmunity against transcriptionally unrepressed target antigen in the thymus of Aire-deficient mice. *J. Immunol.* **174**: 1862–1870.

8. Balandina, A. *et al.* 2005. Functional defect of regulatory CD4⁺CD25⁺ T cells in the thymus of patients with autoimmune myasthenia gravis. *Blood* **105**: 735–741.

9. Masuda, M. *et al.* 2010. Clinical implication of peripheral CD4⁺CD25⁺ regulatory T cells and Th17 cells in myasthenia gravis patients. *J. Neuroimmunol.* **225**: 123–131.

10. Fattorossi, A. *et al.* 2005. Circulating and thymic CD4 CD25 T regulatory cells in myasthenia gravis: effect of immunosuppressive treatment. *Immunology* **116**: 134–141.

11. Sun, Y. *et al.* 2004. Increase of circulating CD4⁺CD25⁺ T cells in myasthenia gravis patients with stability and thymectomy. *Clin. Immunol.* **112**: 284–289.

12. Karube, K. *et al.* 2004. Expression of FoxP3, a key molecule in CD4CD25 regulatory T cells, in adult T-cell leukaemia/lymphoma cells. *Br. J. Haematol.* **126**: 81–84.

13. Luther, C. *et al.* 2005. Decreased frequency of intrathymic regulatory T cells in patients with myasthenia-associated thymoma. *J. Neuroimmunol.* **164**: 124–128.

14. Aricha, R. *et al.* 2008. Ex vivo generated regulatory T cells modulate experimental autoimmune myasthenia gravis. *J. Immunol.* **180**: 2132–2139.

15. Scarpino, S. *et al.* 2007. Expression of autoimmune regulator gene (AIRE) and T regulatory cells in human thymomas. *Clin. Exp. Immunol.* **149**: 504–512.

16. Giraud, M. *et al.* 2007. An IRF8-binding promoter variant and AIRE control CHRNA1 promiscuous expression in thymus. *Nature* **448**: 934–937.

17. Strobel, P. *et al.* 2007. Deficiency of the autoimmune regulator AIRE in thymomas is insufficient to elicit autoimmune polyendocrinopathy syndrome type 1 (APS-1). *J. Pathol.* **211**: 563–571.

18. Kisand, K. *et al.* 2010. Chronic mucocutaneous candidiasis in APECED or thymoma patients correlates with autoimmunity to Th17-associated cytokines. *J. Exp. Med.* **207**: 299–308.

19. Aricha, R. *et al.* 2011. The susceptibility of Aire(−/−) mice to experimental myasthenia gravis involves alterations in regulatory T cells. *J. Autoimmun.* **36**: 16–24.

20. Campbell, I. K. *et al.* 2009. Autoimmune regulator controls T cell help for pathogenetic autoantibody production in collagen-induced arthritis. *Arthritis Rheum.* **60**: 1683–1693.

21. Liston, A. *et al.* 2003. Aire regulates negative selection of organ-specific T cells. *Nat. Immunol.* **4**: 350–354.

22. Aschenbrenner, K. *et al.* 2007. Selection of Foxp3+ regulatory T cells specific for self antigen expressed and presented by Aire+ medullary thymic epithelial cells. *Nat. Immunol.* **8**: 351–358.

23. Hinterberger, M. *et al.* Autonomous role of medullary thymic epithelial cells in central CD4(+) T cell tolerance. *Nat. Immunol.* **11**: 512–519.

24. Gavin, M. A. *et al.* 2007. Foxp3-dependent programme of regulatory T-cell differentiation. *Nature* **445**: 771–775.

25. Wolff, A. S. *et al.* Flow cytometry study of blood cell subtypes reflects autoimmune and inflammatory processes in autoimmune polyendocrine syndrome type I. *Scand. J. Immunol.* **71**: 459–467.

26. Laakso, S. M. *et al.* 2010. Regulatory T cell defect in APECED patients is associated with loss of naive FOXP3(+) precursors and impaired activated population. *J. Autoimmun.* **35**: 351–357.

27. Prelog, M. *et al.* 2009. Thymectomy in early childhood: significant alterations of the CD4(+)CD45RA(+)CD62L(+) T cell compartment in later life. *Clin. Immunol.* **130**: 123–132.

Ann. N.Y. Acad. Sci. ISSN 0077-8923

ANNALS OF THE NEW YORK ACADEMY OF SCIENCES
Issue: *Myasthenia Gravis and Related Disorders*

Pathogenic IgG4 subclass autoantibodies in MuSK myasthenia gravis

Jaap J. Plomp,[1,2] Maartje G. Huijbers,[1,3] Silvère M. van der Maarel,[3] and Jan J. Verschuuren[1]

[1]Department of Neurology, [2]Department of MCB-Neurophysiology, [3]Department of Human Genetics, Medical Genetics Center, Leiden University Medical Center, Leiden, the Netherlands

Address for correspondence: Dr. J. J. Plomp, Ph.D., Leiden University Medical Center, Depts. Neurology and MCB Neurophysiology, Research Building, S5-P, P.O. Box 9600, 2300 RC Leiden, the Netherlands. j.j.plomp@lumc.nl

Autoantibodies against muscle-specific kinase (MuSK), a protein essential for clustering of acetylcholine receptors at the neuromuscular junction (NMJ), are detected in the serum of a proportion of myasthenia gravis (MG) patients. In most MuSK MG patients the anti-MuSK activity resides in the IgG4 subclass, a minor IgG component without very well-defined, but presumably anti-inflammatory, roles in immunity. In recent years, several animal model studies showed that anti-MuSK autoantibodies can cause muscle weakness by directly affecting NMJ function and, therefore, are likely not simply bystander disease markers in MuSK MG patients. In passive transfer mice, we recently provided proof that MuSK MG patient IgG4 is severely myasthenogenic, causing functional defects at NMJs. Against the clinical, serological, and pharmacological background of MuSK MG, here we discuss the MuSK MG animal models generated by our laboratory and others that have been instrumental in elucidating the etiological and pathophysiological roles of anti-MuSK antibodies.

Keywords: MuSK; muscle-specific kinase; neuromuscular junction; myasthenia gravis; electrophysiology; mouse model

Introduction

IgG antibodies against muscle-specific kinase (MuSK) were first discovered in 2001 in the serum of a proportion of patients suffering from "seronegative" myasthenia gravis (MG), which was defined at the time as MG without acetylcholine receptor (AChR) antibodies.[1] In the following years, uncertainty has remained as to whether these anti-MuSK antibodies are the pathogenic factors that cause defective synaptic transmission at the neuromuscular junction (NMJ) or whether they are simply bystander disease markers.[2,3] More recently, a number of passive transfer studies in mice unequivocally pinpointed these patient anti-MuSK antibodies as directly myasthenogenic, and very recent work in our laboratory has provided proof that this pathogenicity resides in the IgG4 subclass.

MuSK and the development and maintenance of AChR clustering at the NMJ

MuSK is a single-pass transmembrane protein that is expressed at the postsynaptic membrane of the NMJ. Its N-terminal extracellular region consists of three immunoglobulin-like domains and one Frizzled-like cysteine-rich domain. The intracellular C-terminal region harbors the tyrosine kinase domain. More details on the structure and function of MuSK can be found in several recent reviews.[3–7] MuSK is crucial for embryonic development as well as adult maintenance of the NMJ. This follows from the observations that MuSK-null mutant mice do not form NMJs[8] and that postnatal removal of MuSK in conditional knockout mice or by RNA interference results in disassembly of these synapses.[9,10] Both the

doi: 10.1111/j.1749-6632.2012.06808.x

Ann. N.Y. Acad. Sci. 1275 (2012) 114–122 © 2012 New York Academy of Sciences.

cytoplasmatic and extracellular parts of MuSK interact with several other synaptic molecules. The most important binding partners currently identified are low-density lipoprotein receptor-related protein-4 (LRP4), another postsynaptic transmembrane protein, and downstream of tyrosine kinase/docking protein-7 (DOK7), an intracellular protein involved in cytoplasmatic coactivation of MuSK. The extracellular region of LRP4 forms a membrane receptor for neurally released agrin.[11,12] Interestingly, very recent studies suggest important bidirectional transsynaptic signaling roles for the extracellular domain of LRP4 in NMJ development (1) as an anterograde signal from the motor nerve terminal that modifies postsynaptic differentiation[13] and (2) as a retrograde signal from the muscle fiber that stimulates formation of presynaptic neurotransmitter release sites on the motor nerve terminal.[14] To these ends, LRP4 fragments may be released into the synaptic cleft by proteolytic shedding.[13] Another relevant binding partner of MuSK is collagen-Q, a basal lamina molecule that, in turn, binds acetylcholinesterase (AChE) in the synaptic cleft. For early embryonic (nerve-independent) AChR clustering, the joint presence of MuSK, LRP4, and DOK7 is required, as it is in later stages when the innervating motor nerve growth cone releases agrin, which binds to LRP4. This results in autophosphorylation of the complexed MuSK, which causes association with a second LRP4-MuSK heterodimer and a DOK7 dimer into a stable multimeric complex with activated tyrosine kinase domains. Through a number of intermediate cytoplasmatic factors, this promotes formation of stabile AChR clusters in the postsynaptic membrane of the NMJ. Anti-MuSK antibodies in MuSK MG are thought to interfere with the AChR cluster maintenance role of MuSK, but the exact mechanism of action has yet to be determined.

MuSK myasthenia gravis

MG is characterized by fatigable muscle weakness due to NMJ malfunction. In the most common form of the disease (∼85% of the patients), the muscle weakness is caused by autoantibodies that target AChRs at the NMJ.[15,16] These autoantibodies cross-link AChRs and activate the complement system, leading to removal of AChRs as well as to damage of the postsynaptic membrane. This leads to secondary loss of voltage-gated Na^+ channels that reside in the troughs of the postsynaptic membrane folding at the NMJ.[17] Together, this produces diminished sensitivity for ACh, causing endplate potentials (EPPs) to become small and an elevated threshold for the initiation of a muscle fiber action potential by the EPP. This severely reduces the safety factor of neuromuscular transmission, causing critical "just-suprathreshold" neuromuscular transmission at many NMJs. In repetitive use of such synapses, transmission becomes increasingly blocked due to the naturally occurring rundown of presynaptic ACh release, which causes depression of the already small EPPs so that they become subthreshold and no longer trigger muscle fiber action potentials. In addition to this population of NMJs with critical transmission, a proportion of the NMJs in severely affected MG muscles possesses such a low AChR density that transmission is permanently blocked.

Classically, the ∼15% of MG patients without detectable AChR antibodies has been termed seronegative. However, since 2001, this proportion has become increasingly smaller with the discovery of (1) anti-MuSK antibodies,[1] (2) antibodies against clustered AChRs, detected in a sensitive cell-based assay,[18] and (3), very recently, antibodies to LRP4.[19–21] These previously "seronegative" MG patient subgroups seem to have different clinical, genetic, and pharmacological characteristics. MuSK MG differs in four important aspects from AChR MG: (1) the anti-MuSK antibodies are predominantly of the IgG4 subclass instead of IgG1 and IgG3 (see below);[22–26] (2) there is a specific HLA haplotype association;[27] (3) muscle weakness is typically restricted to bulbar, neck, and respiratory muscles, with frequent respiratory crises;[28,29] and (4) treatment with cholinesterase inhibitors is often suboptimal or even counterproductive.[28,30]

Early MuSK MG muscle biopsy studies suggested that the anti-MuSK antibodies might rather be bystanders than principal pathogenic factors. In one study of intercostal muscle NMJs of a patient who had a high titer of anti-MuSK antibodies, electrophysiological analysis showed small miniature endplate potentials (MEPPs), an important hallmark of MG. Surprisingly, normal AChR and MuSK intensities were found and only faint IgG deposits could be demonstrated.[31] Another NMJ study of motor point biopsies from biceps brachii muscles from eight Japanese MG patients with MuSK antibodies revealed no clear loss of AChRs or considerable deposition of immune complexes at the NMJs. In only two of nine MuSK MG muscle biopsies investigated, complement deposition was observed.[32] This is in agreement with the anti-MuSK antibodies in patients being of the IgG4 subclass, which is unable to activate complement (see below).

In 2008, a clinical–serological study from our group, in collaboration with an Oxford group, showed that in individual MuSK MG patients there is a correlation between the serum (IgG4) anti-MuSK antibody titer and disease severity. Six patients who had 7–12 serum samples collected during 2.5–13.4 years of clinical follow-up were scored retrospectively for myasthenic disease severity on the basis of their clinical charts. A positive correlation between anti-MuSK-specific IgG4 titer and disease severity was found in five of the six patients. Interestingly, one patient made an anti-MuSK antibody subclass switch from IgG4 to IgG1 while going into clinical remission. Together, these findings strongly indicate that anti-MuSK antibodies are the myasthenogenic factor in certain patients and that the IgG4 subclass is responsible. Recent experimental animal studies have corroborated this notion (see below).

AChE inhibiting compounds are standard and beneficial drugs in AChR MG. The majority of MuSK MG patients, however, does not experience long-term benefit from these drugs and may even experience worsening of myasthenic weakness and cholinergic symptoms of overdosing at normal or moderate dosing.[28,29,33,34] Immunosuppressive treatment seems more successful, as in AChR MG. Recent studies indicate that especially rituximab, a monoclonal antibody that causes B cell depletion, might provide long-term improvement in MuSK MG.[3,35]

IgG4 subclass antibodies

As described above, there are strong indications that anti-MuSK IgG4 is the major culprit in MuSK MG patients. Human IgG comprises four subclasses (IgG1, IgG2, IgG3, and IgG4), each having specific structural and functional characteristics.[36] Several features distinguish IgG4 from the other subclasses:[37] (1) it is the least abundant in serum (<5% of total IgG); (2) it does not activate complement due to its inability to bind to C1q, one of the first components in the complement cascade;[38]

(3) it only weakly binds Fcγ-receptors on immune cells and thus is not a strong activator of such cells; and (4) it can recombine half-antibodies with other IgG4 molecules ("Fab-arm exchange"), leading to hybrid antibodies that are hetero-bispecific and thus do not cross-link antigens.[37,39,40] In view of these characteristics, IgG4 is considered benign and anti-inflammatory. IgG4 possibly offers protection against nonmicrobial antigens after chronic exposure, for example, against bee venom in bee keepers. However, antigen-specific IgG4 is found in a number of autoimmune conditions, including a variant of the skin-blistering disease pemphigus against cell adhesion desmoglein proteins,[41] in idiopathic membranous glomerulonephritis against M-type phospholipase-A2 receptors,[42] and in thrombotic thrombocytopenic purpura against a metalloproteinase ADAMTS13.[43] Of these disorders, pathogenicity of the antigen-specific IgG4 has only been experimentally shown for pemphigus, with passive transfer experiments in mice,[44] although the precise pathological effects are not yet clarified. Recently, our group provided evidence of IgG4 pathogenicity in MuSK MG (see below).

MuSK myasthenia gravis animal models

Active immunization models

Several animal models for MuSK MG have been developed in recent years, most of them based on active immunization of animals with heterologous MuSK (fragments). The first two models were published in 2006.[45–47] Repetitive injection of a chimeric protein composed of the MuSK ectodomain and the Fc region of human IgG1 into rabbits caused paralysis within three to nine weeks.[46] AChR density and area were reduced, and repetitive nerve stimulation electromyography revealed decrementing compound muscle action potentials (CMAPs), all indicative of NMJ dysfunction. The anti-MuSK antibodies produced by these rabbits were further characterized in a cellular assay where they inhibited agrin-dependent and -independent AChR clustering. Similarly, paralysis resulted in mice after two to three injections of a recombinant protein containing the extracellular domain of rat MuSK.[45] Several mouse strains were used. While most B6, A/J, and bm12 mice showed myasthenic weakness after four to eight weeks, BALB/c mice were not responsive, in spite of having low-titer anti-MuSK antibodies, indicating that genetic factors modify the immune response. The weakness was caused by NMJ defects, as demonstrated by CMAP decrement, reduced and fragmented AChR fields in fluorescence microscopy, and reduced MEPP amplitude, indicating a reduced postsynaptic sensitivity for the neurotransmitter ACh. Except for BALB/c serum, the sera of these MuSK MG mice strongly inhibited agrin-induced AChR clustering in C2C12 myocytes in culture. Further characterizations showed that NMJs in so-called fast-synapsing muscles (which form NMJs rapidly during development) are more resistant to damaging effects of the anti-MuSK antibodies than NMJs in delayed synapsing muscle (which form NMJs more slowly during development).[47] This may contribute to the regional muscle differences in susceptibility to weakness in MuSK MG. Another factor may be the variation of intrinsic MuSK levels among different muscles.[48] Interestingly, the MuSK mRNA level in, for example, mouse masseter muscle is low, and this muscle appears to be severely affected, with signs of denervation atrophy, in an active immunization study.[49] Furthermore, while in muscle with a high MuSK mRNA level there is nerve sprouting as a response to the postsynaptic effects of anti-MuSK antibodies at NMJs, muscle with a low MuSK mRNA level does not show such a secondary effect.[49]

Detailed microelectrode studies at diaphragm muscle NMJs of (symptomatic) active immunization MuSK MG mice revealed a reduced MEPP amplitude,[45,50,51] which is compatible with the observed reduced and fragmented AChR field. Of note, there were also changes in presynaptic ACh release parameters. The spontaneous release of ACh quanta, measured as MEPP frequency, was severely reduced.[50,51] In addition, nerve stimulation-evoked release was found either unchanged[51] or reduced,[50] which in both cases can be regarded as a defect, since in myasthenic NMJs there is normally a robust compensatory upregulation of evoked ACh release—the quantal content (i.e., the number of ACh quanta released per nerve impulse).[52] Ultrastructurally, NMJs from symptomatic active immunization MuSK MG mouse and rat models show reduced postsynaptic foldings and nerve terminal segmentation, in line with the fluorescence microscopical observations.[50,53]

Passive immunization models

While the active immunization models have yielded important etiological and pathophysiological infor-

mation, one important drawback is that the anti-MuSK antibodies produced are not of human origin and may thus have different characteristics that affect their pathological mode of action. Besides, one of Witebsky's postulates that must be fulfilled to prove the autoimmune nature of a disease is that symptoms can be reproduced in an experimental animal by direct transfer of the human autoantibody.[54] To this end, several passive transfer studies using MuSK MG patient plasma or purified IgG have recently been undertaken in mice. However, in retrospect, the first study was done already in 1994, when mice were injected with plasma and IgG from seven patients, which were at that time still diagnosed with seronegative MG;[55] later, it appeared that these patients were predominantly seropositive for anti-MuSK antibodies.[56] In the mice, a reduction of MEPP amplitude in diaphragm NMJs was found, without an apparent effect on evoked ACh release, leading to a reduced safety factor of neuromuscular transmission. This was confirmed by increased D-tubocurarine sensitivity of nerve stimulation-induced muscle contraction. Enigmatically, no reduction in AChR number was demonstrated with radioactively labeled α-bungarotoxin. However, in the first passive transfer study in the recent era using purified MuSK MG patient IgGs, AChR reduction was clearly shown by quantitative fluorescence microscopy using fluorescently labeled α-bungarotoxin; the level of AChR reduction was compatible with NMJ dysfunction, which explained the observed muscle weakness and body weight loss.[57] In addition, CMAP decrement was found upon repetitive nerve stimulation. These studies indicated that human MuSK IgG indeed contains the myasthenogenic factor. In further morphological analyses, including fluorescence resonance energy transfer microscopy, AChR density reduction was further substantiated.[58] Interestingly, double-labeling of pre- and postsynaptic elements of the NMJ showed that MuSK MG IgG disturbed the precise alignment between the nerve terminal and the postsynaptic AChR field. In another passive transfer mouse study, MuSK MG IgG was found to severely reduce the basal lamina molecule collagen-Q at NMJs, in conjunction with moderate reduction of AChR and MuSK intensities.[59] Further characterization in an *in vitro* plate-binding assay showed that MuSK MG IgG prevents binding of collagen-Q and MuSK. Because collagen-Q also binds AChE in the synaptic cleft, MuSK MG IgG may reduce the functional expression of this ACh-degrading enzyme. This may explain the unsatisfactory therapeutic effects of AChE inhibitors in MuSK MG. In another passive transfer mouse model, local injection of MuSK MG whole plasma induced subclinical myasthenia in regenerating foot muscle.[60]

In our own laboratory, in passive transfer experiments we have successfully tested the hypothesis that MuSK MG IgG4 is the principal pathogenic factor.[61] We purified MuSK MG IgG4 and IgG1–3 subclass fractions from the plasma of four MuSK MG patients, using high-affinity human IgG subclass-specific ligands, and injected the subclass fractions daily for several weeks into immunodeficient NOD/*scid* mice (preventing immunity against human IgG). IgG4, but not IgG1–3, from the MuSK MG patients induced severe muscle weakness in the mice, starting at approximately one to two weeks depending on the dose and patient origin. Decrements in CMAPs upon repetitive nerve stimulation indicated NMJ dysfunction causing a reduced safety factor of neuromuscular transmission that was confirmed by an increase in D-tubocurarine sensitivity in diaphragm muscle contraction experiments. IgG4 caused reduced density and fragmented area of AChRs and reduced postsynaptic membrane folds at NMJs, similar to the morphological defects observed in active immunization models[45,46,49,50,53] and in the whole-IgG passive transfer mouse model.[57,58] A detailed electrophysiological microelectrode NMJ study revealed severe reduction of MEPP and EPP amplitudes, reduced MEPP frequency, and exaggerated depression of EPPs during physiological, high-rate nerve stimulation. Intriguingly, transmitter release upregulation was lacking, which is the normal homeostatic response in AChR MG. Thus, we demonstrated post- and presynaptic NMJ deficits, explaining the (fatigable) muscle weakness, and proved that MuSK MG IgG4 alone is severely myasthenogenic. These synaptic electrophysiological abnormalities are very similar to those recently reported by an Oxford group for NMJs in whole-IgG MuSK MG passive transfer mice,[51] as well as to those reported by Japanese researchers after active MuSK immunization.[50] A very recent whole-IgG MuSK MG passive transfer study in mice showed that AChR loss begins directly after the start of the daily IgG injections,

progresses more or less linearly at a pace of ~3–4% per day, and is paralleled by a gradual reduction of MEPP amplitude and frequency.[62] This rate of AChR loss matches the rate by which AChRs are inserted at the NMJ during physiological turnover and thus suggests that the initial effect of anti-MuSK IgG is a plain block of insertion of newly synthesized AChRs.

Data from microelectrode studies of NMJs in MuSK MG patient muscle biopsies support these mouse studies: reduced MEPP amplitude without compensatory increased ACh release have been shown,[31,63] paralleled by low MEPP frequency and extra EPP rundown.[63] These similarities impart great clinical relevance to the MuSK MG mouse models. The absence of compensatory increase in ACh release suggests a role for MuSK in synaptic homeostasis (see below).

Drug studies in MuSK myasthenia gravis animal models

Some MuSK MG mouse models have been used to study the response to AChE-inhibiting drugs. The first active immunization mouse study showed that a single i.p. injection of the AChE inhibitor neostigmine partially corrected CMAP amplitude decrements.[45] This was confirmed in a later study,[50] and, in addition, a delayed and fast-decrementing second CMAP—an electromyographical feature of congenital AChE deficiency—was noted.[64] A reduction in AChE staining intensity of ~30% at NMJs and a broadening of EPPs formed further support for the hypothesis that anti-MuSK antibodies indirectly reduce AChE density (possibly by disrupting the interaction between collagen-Q, the AChE anchoring basal lamina protein, and MuSK). In line with this notion, a MuSK MG whole-IgG passive transfer mouse study and another active immunization study, respectively, showed reduction of AChE protein expression at NMJs[59] and reduced AChE mRNA at some muscle types.[49] In the latter model, AChE inhibitor injection also induced delayed, fast-decrementing secondary CMAPs in the gastrocnemius as well as masseter muscles, in addition to fibrillation potentials in the latter muscle, indicative of functional denervation induced by anti-MuSK antibodies. Thus, these animal studies suggest AChE deficiency in MuSK MG patient NMJs. However, AChE was not deficient at the NMJs of intercostal muscle in one MuSK MG patient,[31] and no NMJ electrophysiological evidence of AChE shortage (e.g., broadening of MEPPs and EPPs) has been provided so far in human MuSK MG NMJs.[31,63] It is evident that further studies are needed.

With most MuSK MG patients being hypersensitive to AChE inhibitors, treatment with 3,4-diaminopyridine, successfully used in the treatment of the presynaptic NMJ disorder Lambert-Eaton myasthenic syndrome, might be an alternative drug. In an active MuSK MG immunization mouse model, injection of 3,4-diaminopyridine nearly normalized the CMAP decrement, and *ex vivo* the drug greatly potentiated EPPs in diaphragm NMJs from myasthenic animals.[65]

Pathophysiological mechanisms

Although the recent MuSK MG mouse model studies have provided convincing evidence that anti-MuSK antibodies are principal myasthenogenic factors in the human disease, the exact pathophysiological mechanisms leading to AChR dispersal at the NMJ have yet to be determined. Our own passive transfer study in immunodeficient NOD/*scid* mice provided proof that IgG4 subclass antibodies are the principal responsible factors.[61] This excludes complement-mediated mechanisms, because IgG4 can not activate complement and Nod/scid mice do not have an active complement system.[66] Complement independence has also been indicated by the successful generation of an active MuSK immunization model in complement component C5-deficient mice.[50] The anti-MuSK antibodies evoked in these mice were predominantly of the mouse IgG1 subclass, which shares some characteristics with human IgG4, including the inability to activate complement.[38,50,67] In spite of these experimental findings it cannot be excluded that in some MuSK MG cases, in which some additional anti-MuSK IgG1 or IgG3 is present, pathology involves some degree of complement activation. On the other hand, the example of a MuSK MG patient going into remission while making a subclass switch from IgG4 to IgG1 anti-MuSK antibody argues against the pathogenic relevance of anti-MuSK IgG1.[23] The Fab arm exchange–induced hetero-bivalency of anti-MuSK IgG4 antibodies may be of crucial importance for pathogenic mechanisms. In an elegant first study to elucidate this possibility, IgG from the serum of symptomatic active immunization MuSK MG rabbits was papain-cleaved into Fab fragments, and the effects of whole IgG versus Fab was studied on AChR clustering in C2C12 myotubes in culture.[68] It appeared that both bivalent (the IgG) and monovalent antibodies (the Fab) can inhibit the AChR clustering function of MuSK, via two distinct (hypothesized) mechanisms: bivalent IgG cross-links and activates MuSK molecules by autophosphorylation, and MuSK is then internalized and downregulated; or monovalent Fab, which is unable to cross-link MuSK molecules, directly inhibits autophosphorylation and thereby inhibits activation of MuSK without subsequent internalization. It remains to be seen how this translates to the pathogenic human MuSK MG IgG4. In any case, the balance between the two mechanisms will be determined by the ratio of bi- and monovalent IgG4 present, which in turn depends on the level of Fab arm exchange in the patient *in vivo*. Further studies using human MuSK MG antibodies are needed.

Irrespective of the underlying mechanisms by which anti-MuSK antibodies disturb AChR clustering at NMJs, it is clear from animal model studies and from MuSK MG biopsy analyses that besides postsynaptic changes there are also morphological and functional changes in the presynaptic nerve terminal. A direct action of anti-MuSK IgG on the nerve terminal is unlikely because it presumably contains no MuSK.[69] More likely, postsynaptic loss of MuSK function at the NMJ either directly or indirectly disturbs functional and structural synapse homeostasis mechanisms that normally cause increased presynaptic ACh release in response to postsynaptic AChR loss at NMJs, a process involving unknown retrograde signaling factors.[52,70,71] At NMJs of MuSK MG IgG4–injected myasthenic mice, we observed failure of this important homeostatic response and aggravating weakness. Similarly, the absence of ACh release increase was found at myasthenic NMJs of active immunized mice, as well as NMJs of MuSK MG whole-IgG passive transfer mice.[50,51,62] Together, these studies suggest a crucial role for MuSK in homeostasis, for example, in sensing AChR loss or in releasing retrograde messenger substances. Of note, some MuSK-signaling pathway factors such as agrin and rapsyn are involved with the postsynaptic dystrophin glycoprotein complex,[6,72–74] which is thought to influence NMJ structure, function, and synaptic homeostasis.[73,75] Clearly, further studies are needed to elucidate the complex interplay of MuSK MG IgG4 autoantibodies, MuSK function, and synaptic plasticity at myasthenic NMJs.

Acknowledgments

This work was supported by the Prinses Beatrix Fonds (WAR09-19) and L'Association Française contre les Myopathies (#15363).

Conflicts of interest

The authors declare no conflicts of interest.

References

1. Hoch, W., J. McConville, S. Helms, *et al.* 2001. Autoantibodies to the receptor tyrosine kinase MuSK in patients with myasthenia gravis without acetylcholine receptor antibodies. *Nat. Med.* **7:** 365–368.
2. Lindstrom, J. 2004. Is "seronegative" MG explained by autoantibodies to MuSK? *Neurology* **62:** 1920–1921.
3. Shi, L., A.K. Fu & N.Y. Ip. 2012. Molecular mechanisms underlying maturation and maintenance of the vertebrate neuromuscular junction. *Trends Neurosci.* **35:** 441–453.
4. Ghazanfari, N., K.J. Fernandez, Y. Murata, *et al.* 2011. Muscle specific kinase: organiser of synaptic membrane domains. *Int. J. Biochem. Cell Biol.* **43:** 295–298.
5. Punga, A.R. & M.A. Ruegg. 2012. Signaling and aging at the neuromuscular synapse: lessons learnt from neuromuscular diseases. *Curr. Opin. Pharmacol.* **12:** 340–346.
6. Wu, H., W.C. Xiong & L. Mei. 2010. To build a synapse: signaling pathways in neuromuscular junction assembly. *Development* **137:** 1017–1033.
7. Burden, S.J. 2011. SnapShot: neuromuscular Junction. *Cell* **144:** 826.
8. Dechiara, T.M., D.C. Bowen, D.M. Valenzuela, *et al.* 1996. The receptor tyrosine kinase MuSK is required for neuromuscular junction formation in vivo. *Cell* **85:** 501–512.
9. Kong, X.C., P. Barzaghi & M.A. Ruegg. 2004. Inhibition of synapse assembly in mammalian muscle in vivo by RNA interference. *EMBO Rep.* **5:** 183–188.
10. Hesser, B.A., O. Henschel & V. Witzemann. 2006. Synapse disassembly and formation of new synapses in postnatal muscle upon conditional inactivation of MuSK. *Mol. Cell Neurosci.* **31:** 470–480.
11. Kim, N., A.L. Stiegler, T.O. Cameron, *et al.* 2008. Lrp4 is a receptor for Agrin and forms a complex with MuSK. *Cell* **135:** 334–342.
12. Gomez, A.M. & S.J. Burden. 2011. The extracellular region of Lrp4 is sufficient to mediate neuromuscular synapse formation. *Dev. Dyn.* **240:** 2626–2633.
13. Wu, H., Y. Lu, C. Shen, *et al.* 2012. Distinct roles of muscle and motoneuron LRP4 in neuromuscular junction formation. *Neuron* **75:** 94–107.
14. Yumoto, N., N. Kim & S.J. Burden. 2012. Lrp4 is a retrograde signal for presynaptic differentiation at neuromuscular synapses. *Nature* **489:** 438–442.
15. Farrugia, M.E. & A. Vincent. 2010. Autoimmune mediated neuromuscular junction defects. *Curr. Opin. Neurol.* **23:** 489–495.
16. Verschuuren, J.J., J. Palace & N.E. Gilhus. 2010. Clinical aspects of myasthenia explained. *Autoimmunity* **43:** 344–352.
17. Serra, A., R. Ruff, H. Kaminski & R.J. Leigh. 2011. Factors contributing to failure of neuromuscular transmission in myasthenia gravis and the special case of the extraocular muscles. *Ann. N.Y. Acad. Sci.* **1233:** 26–33.
18. Leite, M.I., S. Jacob, S. Viegas, *et al.* 2008. IgG1 antibodies to acetylcholine receptors in 'seronegative' myasthenia gravis. *Brain* **131:** 1940–1952.
19. Zhang, B., J.S. Tzartos, M. Belimezi, *et al.* 2012. Autoantibodies to lipoprotein-related protein 4 in patients with double-seronegative myasthenia gravis. *Arch. Neurol.* **69:** 445–451.
20. Pevzner, A., B. Schoser, K. Peters, *et al.* 2012. Anti-LRP4 autoantibodies in AChR- and MuSK-antibody-negative myasthenia gravis. *J. Neurol.* **259:** 427–435.
21. Higuchi, O., J. Hamuro, M. Motomura & Y. Yamanashi. 2011. Autoantibodies to low-density lipoprotein receptor-related protein 4 in myasthenia gravis. *Ann. Neurol.* **69:** 418–422.
22. McConville, J., M.E. Farrugia, D. Beeson, *et al.* 2004. Detection and characterization of MuSK antibodies in seronegative myasthenia gravis. *Ann. Neurol.* **55:** 580–584.
23. Niks, E.H., Y. van Leeuwen, M.I. Leite, *et al.* 2008. Clinical fluctuations in MuSK myasthenia gravis are related to antigen-specific IgG4 instead of IgG1. *J. Neuroimmunol.* **195:** 151–156.
24. Ohta, K., K. Shigemoto, A. Fujinami, *et al.* 2007. Clinical and experimental features of MuSK antibody positive MG in Japan. *Eur. J. Neurol.* **14:** 1029–1034.
25. Tsiamalos, P., G. Kordas, A. Kokla, K. Poulas & S.J. Tzartos. 2009. Epidemiological and immunological profile of muscle-specific kinase myasthenia gravis in Greece. *Eur. J. Neurol.* **16:** 925–930.
26. Vincent, A. & J. Newsom-Davis. 1982. Acetylcholine receptor antibody characteristics in myasthenia gravis: I. Patients with generalized myasthenia or disease restricted to ocular muscles. *Clin. Exp. Immunol.* **49:** 257–265.
27. Niks, E.H., J.B. Kuks, B.O. Roep, *et al.* 2006. Strong association of MuSK antibody-positive myasthenia gravis and HLA-DR14-DQ5. *Neurology* **66:** 1772–1774.
28. Evoli, A., P.A. Tonali, L. Padua, *et al.* 2003. Clinical correlates with anti-MuSK antibodies in generalized seronegative myasthenia gravis. *Brain* **126:** 2304–2311.
29. Guptill, J.T., D.B. Sanders & A. Evoli. 2011. Anti-MuSK antibody myasthenia gravis: clinical findings and response to treatment in two large cohorts. *Muscle Nerve* **44:** 36–40.
30. Guptill, J.T. & D.B. Sanders. 2010. Update on muscle-specific tyrosine kinase antibody positive myasthenia gravis. *Curr. Opin. Neurol.* **23:** 530–535.
31. Selcen, D., T. Fukuda, X.M. Shen & A.G. Engel. 2004. Are MuSK antibodies the primary cause of myasthenic symptoms? *Neurology* **62:** 1945–1950.
32. Shiraishi, H., M. Motomura, T. Yoshimura, *et al.* 2005. Acetylcholine receptors loss and postsynaptic damage in MuSK antibody-positive myasthenia gravis. *Ann. Neurol.* **57:** 289–293.

33. Hatanaka, Y., S. Hemmi, M.B. Morgan, *et al.* 2005. Non-responsiveness to anticholinesterase agents in patients with MuSK-antibody-positive MG. *Neurology* **65:** 1508–1509.

34. Punga, A.R., R. Flink, H. Askmark & E.V. Stalberg. 2006. Cholinergic neuromuscular hyperactivity in patients with myasthenia gravis seropositive for MuSK antibody. *Muscle Nerve* **34:** 111–115.

35. Diaz-Manera, J., E. Martinez-Hernandez, L. Querol, *et al.* 2012. Long-lasting treatment effect of rituximab in MuSK myasthenia. *Neurology* **78:** 189–193.

36. Schroeder, H.W., Jr. & L. Cavacini. 2010. Structure and function of immunoglobulins. *J. Allergy Clin. Immunol.* **125:** S41–S52.

37. Aalberse, R.C., S.O. Stapel, J. Schuurman & T. Rispens. 2009. Immunoglobulin G4: an odd antibody. *Clin. Exp. Allergy* **39:** 469–477.

38. Daha, N.A., N.K. Banda, A. Roos, *et al.* 2011. Complement activation by (auto-) antibodies. *Mol. Immunol.* **48:** 1656–1665.

39. Aalberse, R.C. & J. Schuurman. 2002. IgG4 breaking the rules. *Immunology* **105:** 9–19.

40. van der Neut-Kolfschoten M., J. Schuurman, M. Losen, *et al.* 2007. Anti-inflammatory activity of human IgG4 antibodies by dynamic Fab arm exchange. *Science* **317:** 1554–1557.

41. Sitaru, C., S. Mihai & D. Zillikens. 2007. The relevance of the IgG subclass of autoantibodies for blister induction in autoimmune bullous skin diseases. *Arch. Dermatol. Res.* **299:** 1–8.

42. Beck, L.H., Jr., R.G. Bonegio, G. Lambeau, *et al.* 2009. M-type phospholipase A2 receptor as target antigen in idiopathic membranous nephropathy. *N. Engl. J. Med.* **361:** 11–21.

43. Ferrari, S., G.C. Mudde, M. Rieger, *et al.* 2009. IgG subclass distribution of anti-ADAMTS13 antibodies in patients with acquired thrombotic thrombocytopenic purpura. *J. Thromb. Haemost.* **7:** 1703–1710.

44. Rock, B., C.R. Martins, A.N. Theofilopoulos, *et al.* 1989. The pathogenic effect of IgG4 autoantibodies in endemic pemphigus foliaceus (fogo selvagem). *N. Engl. J. Med.* **320:** 1463–1469.

45. Jha, S., K. Xu, T. Maruta, *et al.* 2006. Myasthenia gravis induced in mice by immunization with the recombinant extracellular domain of rat muscle-specific kinase (MuSK). *J. Neuroimmunol.* **175:** 107–117.

46. Shigemoto, K., S. Kubo, N. Maruyama, *et al.* 2006. Induction of myasthenia by immunization against muscle-specific kinase. *J. Clin. Invest.* **116:** 1016–1024.

47. Xu, K., S. Jha, W. Hoch & S.E. Dryer. 2006. Delayed synapsing muscles are more severely affected in an experimental model of MuSK-induced myasthenia gravis. *Neuroscience* **143:** 655–659.

48. Punga, A.R., M. Maj, S. Lin, *et al.* 2011. MuSK levels differ between adult skeletal muscles and influence postsynaptic plasticity. *Eur. J. Neurosci.* **33:** 890–898.

49. Punga, A.R., S. Lin, F. Oliveri, *et al.* 2011. Muscle-selective synaptic disassembly and reorganization in MuSK antibody positive MG mice. *Exp. Neurol.* **230:** 207–217.

50. Mori, S., S. Kubo, T. Akiyoshi, *et al.* 2012. Antibodies against muscle-specific kinase impair both presynaptic and postsy-naptic functions in a murine model of myasthenia gravis. *Am. J. Pathol.* **180:** 798–810.

51. Viegas, S., L. Jacobson, P. Waters, *et al.* 2012. Passive and active immunization models of MuSK-Ab positive myasthenia: electrophysiological evidence for pre and postsynaptic defects. *Exp. Neurol.* **234:** 506–512.

52. Plomp, J.J., G.T. Van Kempen, M.B. De Baets, *et al.* 1995. Acetylcholine release in myasthenia gravis: regulation at single end-plate level. *Ann. Neurol.* **37:** 627–636.

53. Richman, D.P., K. Nishi, S.W. Morell, *et al.* 2012. Acute severe animal model of anti-muscle-specific kinase myasthenia: combined postsynaptic and presynaptic changes. *Arch. Neurol.* **69:** 453–460.

54. Rose, N.R. & C. Bona. 1993. Defining criteria for autoimmune diseases (Witebsky's postulates revisited). *Immunol. Today* **14:** 426–430.

55. Burges, J., A. Vincent, P.C. Molenaar, *et al.* 1994. Passive transfer of seronegative myasthenia gravis to mice. *Muscle Nerve* **17:** 1393–1400.

56. Vincent, A., M.I. Leite, M.E. Farrugia, *et al.* 2008. Myasthenia gravis seronegative for acetylcholine receptor antibodies. *Ann. N.Y. Acad. Sci.* **1132:** 84–92.

57. Cole, R.N., S.W. Reddel, O.L. Gervasio & W.D. Phillips. 2008. Anti-MuSK patient antibodies disrupt the mouse neuromuscular junction. *Ann. Neurol.* **63:** 782–789.

58. Cole, R.N., N. Ghazanfari, S.T. Ngo, *et al.* 2010. Patient autoantibodies deplete postsynaptic muscle-specific kinase leading to disassembly of the ACh receptor scaffold and myasthenia gravis in mice. *J. Physiol.* **588:** 3217–3229.

59. Kawakami, Y., M. Ito, M. Hirayama, *et al.* 2011. Anti-MuSK autoantibodies block binding of collagen Q to MuSK. *Neurology* **77:** 1819–1826.

60. ter Beek, W.P., P. Martinez-Martinez, M. Losen, *et al.* 2009. The effect of plasma from muscle-specific tyrosine kinase myasthenia patients on regenerating endplates. *Am. J. Pathol.* **175:** 1536–1544.

61. Klooster, R., J.J. Plomp, M.G. Huijbers, *et al.* 2012. Muscle-specific kinase myasthenia gravis IgG4 autoantibodies cause severe neuromuscular junction dysfunction in mice. *Brain* **135:** 1081–1101.

62. Morsch, M., S.W. Reddel, N. Ghazanfari, *et al.* 2012. Muscle specific kinase autoantibodies cause synaptic failure through progressive wastage of postsynaptic acetylcholine receptors. *Exp. Neurol.* **237:** 286–295.

63. Niks, E.H., J.B. Kuks, J.H. Wokke, *et al.* 2010. Pre- and postsynaptic neuromuscular junction abnormalities in MuSK myasthenia. *Muscle Nerve* **42:** 283–288.

64. Bestue-Cardiel, M., d.C.-A. Saenz, J.L. Capablo-Liesa, *et al.* 2005. Congenital endplate acetylcholinesterase deficiency responsive to ephedrine. *Neurology* **65:** 144–146.

65. Mori, S., M. Kishi, S. Kubo, *et al.* 2012. 3,4-Diaminopyridine improves neuromuscular transmission in a MuSK antibody-induced mouse model of myasthenia gravis. *J. Neuroimmunol.* **245:** 75–78.

66. Shultz, L.D., P.A. Schweitzer, S.W. Christianson, *et al.* 1995. Multiple defects in innate and adaptive immunologic function in NOD/LtSz-scid mice. *J. Immunol.* **154:** 180–191.

67. Lux, A., S. Aschermann, M. Biburger & F. Nimmerjahn. 2010. The pro and anti-inflammatory activities of immunoglobulin G. *Ann. Rheum. Dis.* **69**(Suppl 1): i92–i96.

68. Mori, S., S. Yamada, S. Kubo, J. Chen, *et al.* 2012. Divalent and monovalent autoantibodies cause dysfunction of MuSK by distinct mechanisms in a rabbit model of myasthenia gravis. *J. Neuroimmunol.* **244**: 1–7.

69. Valenzuela, D.M., T.N. Stitt, P.S. Distefano, *et al.* 1995. Receptor tyrosine kinase specific for the skeletal muscle lineage: expression in embryonic muscle, at the neuromuscular junction, and after injury. *Neuron* **15**: 573–584.

70. Plomp, J.J., G.T. Van Kempen & P.C. Molenaar. 1992. Adaptation of quantal content to decreased postsynaptic sensitivity at single endplates in alpha-bungarotoxin-treated rats. *J. Physiol.* **458**: 487–499.

71. Sons, M.S., N. Busche, N. Strenzke, *et al.* 2006. alpha-Neurexins are required for efficient transmitter release and synaptic homeostasis at the mouse neuromuscular junction. *Neuroscience* **138**: 433–446.

72. Apel, E.D., S.L. Roberds, K.P. Campbell & J.P. Merlie. 1995. Rapsyn may function as a link between the acetylcholine receptor and the agrin-binding dystrophin-associated glycoprotein complex. *Neuron* **15**: 115–126.

73. Pilgram, G.S., S. Potikanond, R.A. Baines, *et al.* 2010. The roles of the dystrophin-associated glycoprotein complex at the synapse. *Mol. Neurobiol.* **41**: 1–21.

74. Strochlic, L., A. Cartaud & J. Cartaud. 2005. The synaptic muscle-specific kinase (MuSK) complex: new partners, new functions. *Bioessays* **27**: 1129–1135.

75. Noakes, P.G., M. Gautam, J. Mudd, *et al.* 1995. Aberrant differentiation of neuromuscular junctions in mice lacking s-laminin/laminin beta 2. *Nature* **374**: 258–262.

Ann. N.Y. Acad. Sci. ISSN 0077-8923

ANNALS OF THE NEW YORK ACADEMY OF SCIENCES

Issue: *Myasthenia Gravis and Related Disorders*

The search for new antigenic targets in myasthenia gravis

Judith Cossins,[1] Katsiaryna Belaya,[1] Katarzyna Zoltowska,[1] Inga Koneczny,[1] Susan Maxwell,[1] Leslie Jacobson,[2] Maria Isabel Leite,[2] Patrick Waters,[2] Angela Vincent,[2] and David Beeson[1]

[1]Nuffield Department of Clinical Neurosciences, Weatherall Institute of Molecular Medicine, John Radcliffe Hospital, Oxford, United Kingdom. [2]Nuffield Department of Clinical Neurosciences, John Radcliffe Hospital, Oxford, United Kingdom

Address for correspondence: Judith Cossins, Nuffield Department of Clinical Neurosciences, Weatherall Institute of Molecular Medicine, John Radcliffe Hospital, Oxford, UK, OX3 9DS. judith.cossins@imm.ox.ac.uk

Around 80% of myasthenia gravis patients have antibodies against the acetylcholine receptor, and 0–60% of the remaining patients have antibodies against the muscle-specific tyrosine kinase, MuSK. Another recently identified antigen is low-density lipoprotein receptor-related protein 4 (Lrp4). To improve the existing assays and widen the search for new antigenic targets, we have employed cell-based assays in which candidate target proteins are expressed on the cell surface of transfected cells and probed with patient sera. These assays, combined with use of myotube cultures to explore the effects of the antibodies, enable us to begin to identify new antigenic targets and test antibody pathogenicity *in vitro*.

Keywords: myasthenia; autoantibodies; AChR; Lrp4; agrin; ColQ; MuSK

Introduction

Approximately 80% of patients with generalized myasthenia gravis (MG) have autoantibodies against the acetylcholine receptor (AChR) measured by radioimmunoprecipitation assay.[1] The AChR is the ligand-gated ion channel that is densely clustered on the postsynaptic membrane at the neuromuscular junction (NMJ) and is responsible for transmitting the signal from motoneuron to muscle. The clustering of the AChR is dependent on the intracellular scaffold protein, receptor aggregating protein at the synapse (Rapsyn).[2] AChR antibodies are predominantly of the IgG1 and IgG3 subclasses and cause severe loss of AChRs via a number of mechanisms, including complement-mediated damage to the postsynaptic membrane,[3] antigenic modulation resulting in receptor endocytosis,[4] and occasionally by direct AChR block.[5,6]

Around 20% of patients, and a higher proportion of those with purely ocular MG, do not have AChR antibodies (seronegative MG, SNMG). A variable proportion of these SNMG patients, ranging from 0–64%,[7–10] have antibodies against the muscle-specific tyrosine kinase (MuSK).[11] The reason for such a wide range is at least partly due to ge-

ographical variation. In Europe MuSK-MG patients are most frequently found in the northern hemisphere within latitudes 30° and 50° N of the equator.[12] Up to 64% of seronegative patients in Italy have been reported as having MuSK antibodies,[10] whereas there have been few reports of MuSK MG patients in more northern countries such as Norway[9] and Poland.[13] MuSK antibodies are predominantly of the noncomplement-fixing IgG4 subclass,[11] and their pathogenic mechanisms are still unclear.

Cell-based assays for antibodies to AChR, MuSK, and Lrp4

MG patient serum is routinely screened for the presence of AChR and MuSK antibodies using a radioimmunoprecipitation assay (RIA). Although this is a quantitative technique, some patients who are negative in these assays will be positive if they are tested for binding to cells expressing clustered AChRs or high densities of MuSK.[14] In this cell-based assay, HEK293 cells are transfected with the target antigen, and 48 hours later the live cells are incubated with diluted MG patient serum. After washing, the presence of bound patient antibody on the

doi: 10.1111/j.1749-6632.2012.06833.x
Ann. N.Y. Acad. Sci. 1275 (2012) 123–128 © 2012 New York Academy of Sciences.

Table 1. ColQ, Agrin, and Lrp4 antibodies in MG

Antigen	Number of patients with antibodies		Number of patients who also have antibodies against:	
	In all MG patients tested $n = 161$ (percent of total)	In seronegative MG patients $n = 73$ (percent of SN)	AChR	MuSK
ColQ	6 (4%)	4 (5.5%)	0	2
Agrin	24 (15%)	11 (15%)	13	0
Lrp4	13 (8%)	6 (8%)	1	6

The sera tested were from patients with known MG, referred from F. Romi (Norway), A. Evoli (Rome), E.H. Niks (the Netherlands), D. Drachmann (Baltimore), and M. Motomura (Japan).

cells is detected using a fluorescent secondary anti-human IgG antibody. Some previously SNMG sera bound to AChR only when the AChR was clustered by including rapsyn in the transfection.[14] In addition, a small number of SNMG patients were weakly positive for binding to MuSK that expresses very strongly on these cells.[14,15]

For the remaining seronegative patients that do not have antibodies detected by the CBAs, the antigenic targets are still largely unknown. A rational approach is to test proteins that are known to have an important function at the NMJ, and that have extracellular domains that would be accessible to antibodies present in the serum. This approach led to the identification of low-density lipoprotein receptor-related protein 4 (Lrp4) as a target in a variable proportion of seronegative MG patients by several groups.[16–18]

Lrp4 is a transmembrane protein that is the receptor for neural agrin, and it is crucial for the formation and maintenance of the neuromuscular junction.[19–22] Lrp4 antibodies are highly variable in the previous reports, ranging from 3–50%. This wide range is probably a reflection of the fact that several different techniques have been employed. Quantitative methods such as enzyme-linked immunosorbent assays and luciferase assays have been used by some groups to successfully detect antibodies in MG patients.[16,17] However, we favor the semiquantitative cell-based approach in which the glycosylated protein is expressed on the surface of

cells and will adopt a physiological conformation. It will also be expressed at high levels, thus improving detection of antibodies that may bind preferentially to clustered antigens (see Vincent *et al.*[38] for a discussion about the advantages of cell-based assays). Using this cell-based assay, we have detected Lrp4 antibodies in 8% of AChR/MuSK-Ab negative patients (Table 1), but we also detected Lrp4 antibodies in patients with very high levels of MuSK-antibodies, although rarely in any AChR-Ab MG patients.

Other potential antigenic targets

Other potential antigenic targets that are important in NMJ formation or function include neural agrin (Z^+ agrin) and ColQ. Z^+ agrin is an alternatively spliced form of agrin that is specifically released by motoneurons and has up to a 1000-fold greater AChR clustering activity compared with other Z-isoforms.[23] It binds to Lrp4,[19–21] which then activates MuSK, triggering a cascade of events that culminate in the clustering of AChRs on the postsynaptic membrane. ColQ is part of the acetylcholinesterase (AChE) enzyme complex that hydrolyzes acetylcholine and thereby rapidly terminates impulse transmission. ColQ comprises three identical subunits, and it anchors the complex in the synaptic basal lamina.[24] Agrin and ColQ are both present in the synaptic cleft and are therefore accessible to autoantibodies *in vivo*. Moreover, mutations that cause congenital myasthenia syndromes (CMS)

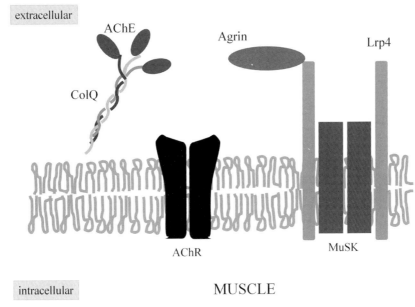

Figure 1. Selection of potential antigenic targets. Schematic diagram showing the key proteins located at the neuromuscular junction.

have been found in both of these proteins,[25–31] and we therefore hypothesized that antibodies against either protein could potentially cause a disturbance of neuromuscular transmission. A schematic diagram showing the location of these and other key proteins at the NMJ is shown in Figure 1.

We used cell-based assays to screen sera from seronegative and seropositive MG patients for antibodies against agrin and ColQ. As ColQ is a secreted protein, we created a DNA construct that expresses ColQ with a transmembrane (TM) domain from contactin-associated protein 2 (Caspr2) fused to its carboxyl terminus. A similar approach has been used for LGI1 antibodies in patients with limbic encephalitis[32] (and see Vincent *et al.*[38]). When HEK293 cells are transfected with this construct ColQ is not secreted but is tethered to the plasma membrane. For the agrin assay we used a similar approach, fusing the secreted form of neural agrin[33] that contains the exons important

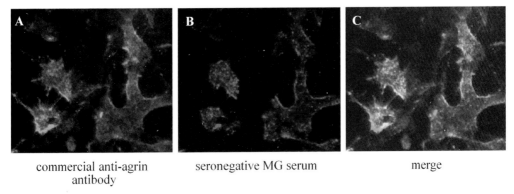

Figure 2. A recombinant form of secreted neural agrin with a C-terminal Caspr2 transmembrane domain is expressed on the surface of HEK293 cells. Transfected cells were incubated with a commercial anti-agrin antibody that was visualized using a green fluorescent secondary antibody (A), or with serum from an MG patient followed by a red fluorescent antibody (B). Commercial antibody and patient serum colocalize (C).

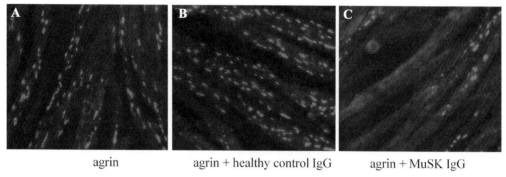

agrin   agrin + healthy control IgG   agrin + MuSK IgG

Figure 3. Functional assay to analyze the effects of autoantibodies from MG patients on AChR clustering *in vitro*. C2C12 myotubes are incubated overnight with a secreted form of neural agrin. Clusters of AChR are visualized with fluorescent α-bungarotoxin (A). Incubation with agrin in the presence of IgG from a healthy control does not affect clustering (B), whereas IgG from an MuSK-MG patient has a negative effect on AChR clustering (C).

for clustering the AChR, with the carboxyl-terminal Caspr2. Agrin is expressed on the surface of HEK293 cells transfected with this construct, as demonstrated using a commercial anti-agrin antibody and fluorescent secondary antibody (Fig. 2A). An example of MG patient serum that recognizes agrin is shown in Figure 2B. The serum staining does not precisely colocalize with the commercial anti-agrin antibody (Fig. 2C), but control-transfected cells (transfected with ColQ or Lrp4) do not stain with patient serum, indicating that the staining is agrin specific. A possible explanation for this discrepancy is that the commercial antibody might recognize different epitopes to the patient serum, and such epitopes might be differentially exposed across the cell surface depending on the conformation of each agrin molecule. Conformation of agrin might also determine the extent to which secondary antibodies can access the relevant primary antibodies. Our preliminary data indicate that antibodies against both agrin and ColQ exist in MG patients (Table 1).

Functional studies using MG sera

Lrp4 is part of the agrin–Lrp4–MuSK–Dok7 pathway that leads to AChR clustering. This pathway can be mimicked *in vitro* using the C2C12 muscle cell line: C2C12 myoblasts are differentiated into myotubes, after which AChR clusters are induced using a soluble form of neural agrin. Agrin-induced AChR clusters are visualized using fluorescent α-bungarotoxin (Fig. 3). The effect of patient serum on AChR clustering can be determined by adding the

serum with the agrin. Using this technique, MuSK antibodies have been shown to alter AChR clustering *in vitro*[34] (Fig. 3C). So far, we have not been able to detect any significant effect on AChR clustering by Lrp4-positive serum from one MG patient using this agrin-induced clustering assay. However, others have used this experimental setup to show that some, but not all, of their Lrp4-positive sera reduce AChR clustering.[17,18] It seems likely therefore that there are differential effects of Lrp4 antibodies. Lrp4 also binds to MuSK, but to date the effect of Lrp4 autoantibodies on this interaction has not been reported. It is also possible that Lrp4 autoantibodies could mediate their effect on the recently described retrograde signalling function of Lrp4.[35] A different experimental setup involving cocultures of motoneurons and myotubes would be required to investigate this.

Agrin promotes the clustering of AChR when applied to myotubes in culture, and we therefore plan to use our *in vitro* AChR clustering assay to investigate the pathogenicity of agrin antibodies. For ColQ antibodies this assay may not be suitable. ColQ anchors AChE complex to the basal lamina. It has been reported to interact with MuSK,[36] but its influence on AChR clustering is unclear. A recent report indicates that MuSK antibodies from one patient that disrupt MuSK-ColQ interaction had a moderate effect on AChR clustering.[37] However, we cannot detect the presence of AChE on myotubes but have not specifically looked for ColQ; this needs to be done. If ColQ is not expressed on C2C12 myotubes, it is unlikely antibodies to this protein will affect AChR clustering, and other experimental approaches will be required to investigate the pathogenicity of ColQ antibodies.

Summary

In summary, we and others are using cell-based assays to screen for new antigenic targets in seronegative MG patients. Cell-based assays have several advantages over RIAs, mainly that the protein is expressed in a native, correctly folded, glycosylated, and physiologically functional state on an intact membrane of a live cell. Antibodies detected by this approach are likely to be pathogenic since they bind to extracellular domains, but further *in vitro* and *in vivo* studies are needed to confirm their pathogenicity. When DNA clones for the proteins are available the cell-based assays are relatively simple to establish. Although time consuming to perform, in the future these assays are likely to provide the gold standard for comparison with other antibody assays, even those that are less labor intensive.

Acknowledgments

We are very grateful to Drs. F. Romi (Norway), A. Evoli (Rome), E.H. Niks (the Netherlands), D. Drachmann (Baltimore), and Dr. M. Motomura (Japan) for use of their sera from MG patients.

Conflicts of interest

The authors declare no conflicts of interest.

References

1. Lang, B. & A. Vincent. 2009. Autoimmune disorders of the neuromuscular junction. *Curr. Opin. Pharmacol.* **9:** 336–340.
2. Phillips, W.D. *et al.* 1991. ACh receptor-rich membrane domains organized in fibroblasts by recombinant 43-kildalton protein. *Science* **251:** 568–570.
3. Engel, A.G. 1984. Myasthenia gravis and myasthenic syndromes. *Ann. Neurol.* **16:** 519–534.
4. Heinemann, S. *et al.* 1977. Modulation of acetylcholine receptor by antibody against the receptor. *Proc. Natl. Acad. Sci. USA* **74:** 3090–3094.
5. Weinberg, C.B. & Z.W. Hall. 1979. Antibodies from patients with myasthenia gravis recognize determinants unique to extrajunctional acetylcholine receptors. *Proc. Natl. Acad. Sci. USA* **76:** 504–508.
6. Burges, J. *et al.* 1990. A myasthenia gravis plasma immunoglobulin reduces miniature endplate potentials at human endplates in vitro. *Muscle Nerve* **13:** 407–413.
7. Sanders, D.B. *et al.* 2003. Clinical aspects of MuSK antibody positive seronegative MG. *Neurology* **60:** 1978–1980.
8. Hoch, W. *et al.* 2001. Auto-antibodies to the receptor tyrosine kinase MuSK in patients with myasthenia gravis without acetylcholine receptor antibodies. *Nat. Med.* **7:** 365–368.
9. Romi, F., J.A. Aarli & N.E. Gilhus. 2005. Seronegative myasthenia gravis: disease severity and prognosis. *Eur. J. Neurol.* **12:** 413–418.
10. Scuderi, F. *et al.* 2002. Anti-p110 autoantibodies identify a subtype of "seronegative" myasthenia gravis with prominent oculobulbar involvement. *Lab. Invest.* **82:** 1139–1146.
11. McConville, J. *et al.* 2004. Detection and characterization of MuSK antibodies in seronegative myasthenia gravis. *Ann. Neurol.* **55:** 580–584.
12. Vincent, A. 2008. Autoantibodies in neuromuscular transmission disorders. *Ann. Indian Acad. Neurol.* **11:** 140–145.
13. Kostera-Pruszczyk, A. *et al.* 2008. MuSK-positive myasthenia gravis is rare in the Polish population. *Eur. J. Neurol.* **15:** 720–724.
14. Leite, M.I. *et al.* 2008. IgG1 antibodies to acetylcholine receptors in 'seronegative' myasthenia gravis. *Brain* **131:** 1940–1952.
15. Jacob, S. *et al.* 2012. Presence and pathogenic relevance of antibodies to clustered acetylcholine receptor in ocular and generalized myasthenia gravis clustered AChR antibodies in myasthenia gravis. *Arch. Neurol.* **69:** 994–1001.
16. Higuchi, O. *et al.* 2011. Autoantibodies to low-density lipoprotein receptor-related protein 4 in myasthenia gravis. *Ann. Neurol.* **69:** 418–422.
17. Zhang, B. *et al.* 2012. Autoantibodies to lipoprotein-related protein 4 in patients with double-seronegative myasthenia gravis. *Arch. Neurol.* **69:** 445–451.
18. Pevzner, A. *et al.* 2012. Anti-LRP4 autoantibodies in AChR- and MuSK-antibody-negative myasthenia gravis. *J. Neurol.* **259:** 427–435.
19. Kim, N. *et al.* 2008. Lrp4 is a receptor for Agrin and forms a complex with MuSK. *Cell* **135:** 334–342.
20. Zhang, B. *et al.* 2008. LRP4 serves as a coreceptor of agrin. *Neuron* **60:** 285–297.
21. Zhang, W. *et al.* 2011. Agrin binds to the N-terminal region of Lrp4 protein and stimulates association between Lrp4 and the first immunoglobulin-like domain in muscle-specific kinase (MuSK). *J. Biol. Chem.* **286:** 40624–40630.
22. Gomez, A.M. & S.J. Burden. 2011. The extracellular region of Lrp4 is sufficient to mediate neuromuscular synapse formation. *Dev. Dyn.* **240:** 2626–2633.
23. Gesemann, M., A.J. Denzer & M.A. Ruegg. 1995. Acetylcholine receptor-aggregating activity of agrin isoforms and mapping of the active site. *J. Cell. Biol.* **128:** 625–636.
24. Peng, H.B. *et al.* 1999. Acetylcholinesterase clustering at the neuromuscular junction involves perlecan and dystroglycan. *J. Cell. Biol.* **145:** 911–921.
25. Wargon, I. *et al.* 2012. Long-term follow-up of patients with congenital myasthenic syndrome caused by COLQ mutations. *Neuromuscul. Disord.* **22:** 318–324.
26. Muller, J.S. *et al.* 2004. Synaptic congenital myasthenic syndrome in three patients due to a novel missense mutation (T441A) of the COLQ gene. *Neuropediatrics* **35:** 183–189.
27. Maselli, R.A. *et al.* 2012. LG2 agrin mutation causing severe congenital myasthenic syndrome mimics functional characteristics of non-neural (z-) agrin. *Hum. Genet.* **131:** 1123–1135.

28. Schreiner, F. *et al.* 2007. Novel COLQ mutation 950delC in synaptic congenital myasthenic syndrome and symptomatic heterozygous relatives. *Neuromuscul. Disord.* **17:** 262–265.
29. Donger, C. *et al.* 1998. Mutation in the human acetylcholinesterase-associated collagen gene, COLQ, is responsible for congenital myasthenic syndrome with end-plate acetylcholinesterase deficiency (Type Ic). *Am. J. Hum. Genet.* **63:** 967–975.
30. Ohno, K. *et al.* 1999. Congenital end-plate acetylcholinesterase deficiency caused by a nonsense mutation and an A–>G splice-donor-site mutation at position +3 of the collagenlike-tail-subunit gene (COLQ): how does G at position +3 result in aberrant splicing? *Am. J. Hum. Genet.* **65:** 635–644.
31. Guven, A., M. Demirci & B. Anlar. 2012. Recurrent COLQ mutation in congenital myasthenic syndrome. *Pediatr. Neurol.* **46:** 253–256.
32. Irani, S.R. *et al.* 2010. Antibodies to Kv1 potassium channel-complex proteins leucine-rich, glioma inactivated 1 protein and contactin-associated protein-2 in limbic encephali-tis, Morvan's syndrome and acquired neuromyotonia. *Brain* **133:** 2734–2748.
33. Hopf, C. & W. Hoch. 1997. Heparin inhibits acetylcholine receptor aggregation at two distinct steps in the agrin-induced pathway. *Eur. J. Neurosci.* **9:** 1170–1177.
34. Farrugia, M.E. *et al.* 2007. Effect of sera from AChR-antibody negative myasthenia gravis patients on AChR and MuSK in cell cultures. *J. Neuroimmunol.* **185:** 136–144.
35. Yumoto, N., N. Kim & S.J. Burden. 2012. Lrp4 is a retrograde signal for presynaptic differentiation at neuromuscular synapses. *Nature* **489:** 438–442.
36. Cartaud, A. *et al.* 2004. MuSK is required for anchoring acetylcholinesterase at the neuromuscular junction. *J. Cell. Biol.* **165:** 505–515.
37. Kawakami, Y. *et al.* 2011. Anti-MuSK autoantibodies block binding of collagen Q to MuSK. *Neurology* **77:** 1819–1826.
38. Vincent, A., P. Waters, M.I. Leite, L. Jacobson, I. Koneczny, J. Cossins & D. Beeson. 2012. Antibodies identified by cell-based assays in myasthenia gravis and associated diseases. *Ann. N.Y. Acad. Sci.* **1274:** 92–98.

Ann. N.Y. Acad. Sci. ISSN 0077-8923

ANNALS OF THE NEW YORK ACADEMY OF SCIENCES
Issue: *Myasthenia Gravis and Related Disorders*

Neuromuscular transmission failure in myasthenia gravis: decrement of safety factor and susceptibility of extraocular muscles

Alessandro Serra,[1] Robert L. Ruff,[2] and Richard John Leigh[2]

[1]Mellen Center for Multiple Sclerosis, Department of Neurology, Cleveland Clinic Foundation, Cleveland, Ohio. [2]Neurology Service, Louis Stokes Veterans Affairs Medical Center, and Case Medical Center, Cleveland, Ohio

Address for correspondence: Alessandro Serra, Mellen Center for Multiple Sclerosis, Cleveland Clinic Foundation, 1950 East 89th Street, Cleveland, Ohio 44195. serraa@ccf.org

An appropriate density of acetylcholine receptors (AChRs) and Na$^+$ channels (NaChs) in the normal neuromuscular junction (NMJ) determines the magnitude of safety factor (SF) that guarantees fidelity of neuromuscular transmission. In myasthenia gravis (MG), an overall simplification of the postsynaptic folding secondary to NMJ destruction results in AChRs and NaChs depletion. Loss of AChRs and NaChs accounts, respectively, for 59% and 40% reduction of the SF at the endplate, which manifests as neuromuscular transmission failure. The extraocular muscles (EOM) have physiologically less developed postsynaptic folding, hence a lower baseline SF, which predisposes them to dysfunction in MG and development of fatigue during "high performance" eye movements, such as saccades. However, saccades in MG show stereotyped, conjugate initial components, similar to normal, which might reflect preserved neuromuscular transmission fidelity at the NMJ of the fast, pale global fibers, which have better developed postsynaptic folding than other extraocular fibers.

Keywords: safety factor; extraocular muscles; saccades; neuromuscular junction

Introduction

In myasthenia gravis (MG), the autoimmune attack is directed toward the acetylcholine receptors (AChRs) at the endplate with consequent complement-mediated destruction of the neuromuscular junction (NMJ). Approximately 50% of patients with MG present with ocular symptoms at onset, while up to 80% develop them during the course of the disease. Several contributing factors might explain the common extraocular muscle (EOM) involvement in MG, including an intrinsic deficiency in complement-inhibitory proteins.[1] Here,[a] we summarize evidence from our previous studies on the role of safety factor reduction at the "myasthenic" NMJ and provide an explanation for some characteristic eye movement findings in MG.[2,3]

Role of the safety factor in the normal neuromuscular junction

In skeletal muscles, the normal postsynaptic architecture consisting of well-developed primary and secondary folding is instrumental in guaranteeing fidelity of neuromuscular transmission. Thus, acetylcholine receptors (AChRs) are more

---

[a]Portions of this paper have been previously published: Serra, A., R. Ruff, H. Kaminski & R.J. Leigh. 2011. Factors contributing to failure of neuromuscular transmission in myasthenia gravis and the special case of the extraocular muscles. *Ann. N.Y. Acad. Sci.* **1233:** 26–33; Otero-Millan, J., S.L. Macknik, A. Serra, R.J. Leigh & S. Martinez-Conde. 2011. Triggering mechanisms in microsaccade and saccade generation: a novel proposal. *Ann. N.Y. Acad. Sci.* **1233:** 107–116; King, S.A., R.M. Schneider, A. Serra & R.J. Leigh. 2011. Critical role of cerebellar fastigial nucleus in programming sequences of saccades. *Ann. N.Y. Acad. Sci.* **1233:** 155–161.

doi: 10.1111/j.1749-6632.2012.06841.x

concentrated at the crest of the primary synaptic folds while the secondary synaptic folds house most of the voltage-gated Na$^+$ channels (NaChs). Following acetylcholine release from the synaptic vesicles in the synaptic space and its consequent binding to the AChRs, channel pores open up generating a localized potential, which results in a current conveyed toward the depths of the secondary synaptic folds where, in turn, the NaChs rapidly open up.[4–8] The passage of the Na$^+$ current through the NaChs ultimately allows the muscle fiber to depolarize. The efficiency of neuromuscular transmission at the skeletal NMJ largely depends on the presence of a safety factor (SF) that ensures that an action potential (AP) is always triggered following acetylcoline release. The SF can be defined by using the formula EPP/E_{AP}, where EPP is the endplate potential amplitude and E_{AP} is the voltage difference between the resting potential (RP) and the action potential threshold.[2] Appropriate concentrations of AChRs and NaChs directly influence the SF magnitude. Thus, while the density of AChRs located at the primary postsynaptic folds increases the size of the EPP, the density of NaChs located at the secondary postsynaptic folds reduces the AP threshold, both ultimately resulting in increased SF magnitude.[2] Direct evidence for the critical role of endplate NaChs in determining an appropriate SF magnitude comes from electrophysiological studies. Thus, the values for E_{AP} and the SF are, respectively, higher and lower at the extrajunctional membrane, where the NaChs are physiologically less concentrated than at the endplate. It is estimated that the NaChs concentration at the endplate directly accounts for 34% of the safety factor.[2]

Decrement of the safety factor at the myasthenic junction

The AChRs antibodies involved in MG directly reduce the number of the endplate AChRs following a combination of complement-mediated membrane lysis and acceleration of AChR catabolism by receptor cross-linking.[9–13] In addition, the voltage-gated NaChs are also depleted as a result of the overall simplification of the postsynaptic folding system that takes place in the disease.[14–16] Experimental models of MG, induced by immunization with foreign or self-AChRs (EAMG) or by passive transfer of myasthenogenic AChR-binding IgG

(PTMG) in the rat, show that the combined loss of AChRs and NaChs results in a direct reduction of the endplate Na$^+$ current at the muscle fibers.[14,17–21]

Loss of AChRs and NaChs account for decreased SF in myasthenia

Here we summarize evidence from our prior studies that the diminished number of endplate AChRs and NaChs in myasthenia directly reduce the SF magnitude,[2] which leaves an exiguous reserve for optimal neuromuscular transmission under demanding conditions (e.g., during exercise), leading to fatigue. The relative impact of AChRs versus NaChs loss in causing decrement of the endplate safety factor was investigated in human myasthenic fibers.[2] Intercostal muscle fibers type IIb were donated by five male patients with myasthenia gravis (age 35–47 years) at the time of thymectomy. All patients had moderately severe generalized myasthenia gravis (MGFA class IIIa) and were seropositive for AChR binding antibodies. Seven control male subjects (age 35–52 years) with no evidence of neuromuscular disease donated control intercostal muscle fibers at the time of a thoracotomy for treatment of cardiac or pulmonary disease. The protocol was approved by the Institutional Review Board of the Department of Veterans Affairs Medical Center in Cleveland. Resting potentials (RPs) in the human intercostal muscle fibers at the endplate and membrane potentials on extrajunctional membrane were measured using intracellular microelectrodes. Miniature endplate potentials (MEPPs) and endplate potentials (EPPs) were similarly measured at the endplate border. Action potential (AP) thresholds were measured using two microelectrodes, one to record the passing current and the other to record the membrane potential.

As expected, RPs were similar for control and MG patients. Both the MEPPs and the EPPs were reduced in fibers from patients with MG, being, respectively, 53% and 58% of the control value. The similar fractional reduction of MEPPs and EPPs is consistent with the notion that reduction in the EPP is due to decrease in the sensitivity of the postsynaptic membrane to acetylcholine. For control human muscle fibers, the depolarization threshold for initiating an AP was lower on the endplate border compared to the extrajunctional membrane, indicating that the density of NaChs was greater at the endplate. The values for AP threshold (E_{AP}) measured on the extrajunctional membrane were similar for MG patients and controls. In contrast, the depolarization needed to trigger an action potential at the endplate was 13.5 mV for controls and 21.6 mV for MG patients.

Ultimately, the safety factor in the type IIb intercostal fibers from MG patients was only 37% of the safety factor in the control fibers, which was equal to 3. Comparison of EPP and E_{AP} values between MG and control fibers made it possible to determine the relative impact on the SF magnitude of diminished number of AChRs and of NaChs. If the EPP of the MG fibers were the same as those of the control fibers, the safety factor for the MG fibers would have been 1.86 rather than the observed value of 1.09. If the E_{AP} of MG fibers were the same as those of the control fibers, the safety factor for the MG fibers would have been 1.74. Thus, the reduction in EPP, which reflects the decreased concentration of AChRs, and the increase in E_{AP}, which reflects the decreased concentration of NaChs, accounted, respectively, for 59% and 40% of the safety factor decrement in skeletal muscle fibers of patients with myasthenia.

In this study, the issue of whether anti-AChRs antibodies in MG reduce Na^+ current at the endplate by a direct action toward the endplate NaChs was also addressed.[2,3] It has been previously established that the gating properties of NaChs away from the endplate are not altered in myasthenia gravis or PTMG, and that, therefore, pathogenic antibodies in myasthenia gravis or PTMG do not target extrajunctional NaChs.[14] Light microscopy and single channel Na^+ current recording techniques were combined to study omohyoid nerve–muscle preparations from rats injected with monoclonal myasthenogenic IgG (McAb3) and inactive antibodies (McAb1), and from control rats. Injecting rats with the inactive McAb1 did not alter Na^+ current at the endplate or on extrajunctional membrane compared with recordings from animals injected with no antibody. Currents recorded from the endplates of rat fibers injected with McAb3 and from rat fibers injected with McAb1 were similar to those recorded from the endplates of rats not treated with an antibody. Thus, rather than by direct impairment, anti-AchRs antibodies cause NaChs dysfunction through complement-mediated destruction of the endplate membrane.[2]

Suceptibility of extraocular muscles in myasthenia

Different structural and functional aspects of the extraocular muscles (EOM) need to be considered in order to explain their common involvement in myasthenia: (1) The EOM and orbital tissue, in general, are intrinsically deficient in complement-inhibitory proteins, being therefore at risk for complement-mediated attack, as it happens in the typical immunological scenario of myasthenia gravis.[1] (2) The EOM are physiologically subject to unusual demands imposed by the visual system, which require sustained and precise ocular alignment for single, binocular vision, in all conditions. Thus, even mild fatigue of the EOM can cause dramatic visual symptoms such as diplopia, whereas similar fatigue of skeletal muscle may be asymptomatic. (3) There are six types of neuromuscular junction fibers identified in the orbital and the global layers of the EOM (Fig. 1). Five of these fibers, whether singly or multiply innervated, lack the well-developed postsynaptic folding system that guarantees an appropriate safety factor and fidelity of neuromuscular transmission in regular skeletal muscles.[22] In other words, EOM fibers are physiologically disadvantaged as the lack of a prominent postsynaptic folding system may result into an inherently lower safety factor, hence increased susceptibility to exercise-induced transmission failure in MG. However, the pale global singly innervated fibers (PGSF) are an exception, as they indeed possess well-developed postsynaptic folding (Fig. 1G). These fibers, which have fast-twitch properties and low fatigue resistance, are believed to briefly discharge at the beginning of a fast (saccadic) eye movement and provide the initial necessary drive to move the eyes toward the desired target.[23]

Dynamics of saccades in ocular myasthenia

Here, we summarize the evidence from our earlier studies to support the hypothesis that the PGSF are relatively spared in ocular myasthenia because of their structural characteristics, which, in turn, accounts for some typical eye movement findings.[3] We studied interocular conjugacy (i.e., how well the eyes move together) of fast eye movements (saccades) from a group of patients affected by ocular myasthenia. As previously shown, interocular conjugacy

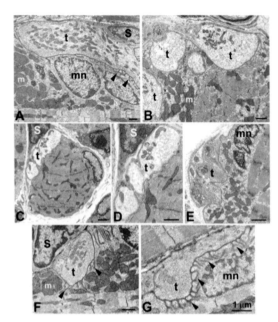

Figure 1. Electron photomicrographs of mouse extraocular muscle neuromuscular junction (NMJ) types. (A and B) Orbital singly innervated fiber (SIF) NMJs encircle individual myofibers, with long terminals (t) embedded in deep depressions of the myofiber surface. Terminals are capped by Schwann cells (S). Postjunctional folding is either absent or sparse (arrowheads), and postjunctional accumulations of myonuclei (mn) and mitochondria (m) are evident. Multiply innervated fiber (MIF) NMJs are small and do not lie in sarcolemmal depressions for both orbital (C and D) and global (E) fiber types. The range of variability in global SIF NMJs includes most junctions with few or no folds (F), but junctions with a high density of postjunctional folds (G) are found, primarily on the global pale SIF type. Reproduced, with permission from Khanna and Porter, *Invest. Ophthalmol. Vis. Sci.* **44:** 1918–1926.

of horizontal saccades in patients with myasthenia gravis affected by disturbance of horizontal gaze was consistently preserved in the initial portion of the eye movement, despite the later component being markedly and variably dysconjugate.[24,25] This was in contrast to consistent normal conjugacy of saccades made by control subjects and abnormal conjugacy of saccades made by patients with lesions at a site other than the NMJ (i.e., abducense nerve palsy or internuclear ophthalmoparesis),[25] who showed instead early and sustained interocular dysconjugacy. However, a minimal dysconjugacy of horizontal saccades exists even in normal subjects, due the physiological delay of signal transmission imposed by the presence of the medial longitudinal fasciculus (MLF) between one set of burst neurons

and one group of motoneurons for the medial rectus muscle.[26,27] Thus, in a later study we focused on vertical saccades in patients with myasthenia gravis who showed disturbances of vertical gaze; in healthy people vertical saccades are tightly yoked (burst neurons in the midbrain rostral interstitial nucleus of the medial longitudinal fasciculus directly project to motoneurons innervating yoke muscle pairs).

In particular, we recorded horizontal and vertical saccades from six patients with MG (age range 40–73 years; median 63), three age-matched patients with cranial nerve palsies (1 oculomotor, 1 trochlear, 1 abducens) and 10 age-matched control subjects. All patients and control subjects gave informed written consent in accordance with the Declaration of Helsinki and the Institutional Review Board of the Cleveland Veterans Affairs Medical Center. On clinical examination of patients with MG, in three cases dysconjugate saccades were evident horizontally; in two cases dysconjugate saccades were evident both horizontally and vertically; and in one case saccades were dysconjugate vertically. During the experimental protocol, subjects viewed a laser spot projected onto a tangent screen at 1.2 m. Saccades were tested as the visual target jumped at 0.25 Hz with amplitude ranging 5–40° horizontally and 5–20° vertically; the direction of target jumps was nonpredictable. Binocular eye movements were recorded using the magnetic search coil technique; coil signals were filtered (0–150 Hz) before digitization at 500 Hz; eye velocity and acceleration were computed as previously described.[28] The interocular conjugacy of horizontal and vertical saccades was assessed using the binocular phase-plane technique.[25] For each saccade, the displacement (change in position) and velocity of each eye were normalized by assigning a value of 1.0 to the maximum displacement and to the peak velocity of the eye making the larger movement. Thus, the phase plane plotted the normalized velocity of each eye against the normalized displacement in 1% (0.01) position increments; this way, we were able to compare the velocity of each eye for the same normalized eye displacement during the entire saccadic movement as a velocity dysconjugacy plot. We applied this technique to over a thousand saccades from the 10 age-matched normal subjects and used linear regression to define 5–95% prediction intervals (PIs). Finally, for each patient, the average velocity dysconjugacy was calculated from at least

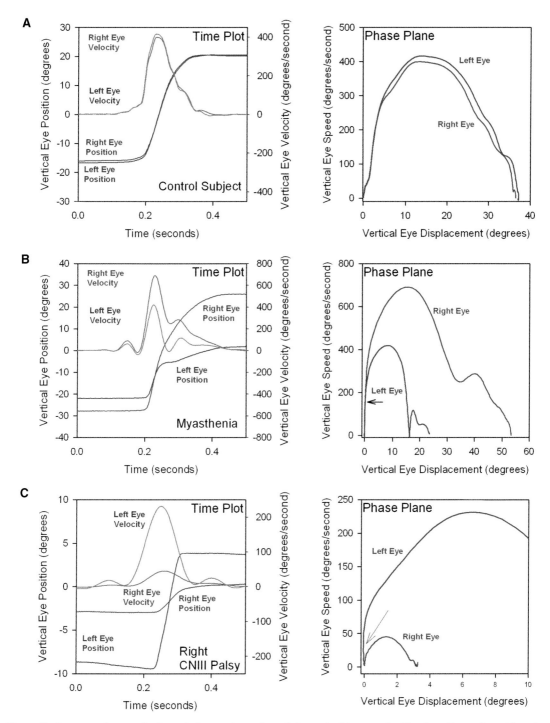

Figure 2. Representative records of a vertical upward saccade made by one healthy control subject (row A), a patient with ocular myasthenia manifest as left pseudo-oculomotor nerve palsy (row B), and a patient with right oculomotor nerve palsy (row C). Each row comprises a time plot of the upward saccade (left panel) and the correspondent phase plane (right panel). The normal subject shows tight interocular saccadic conjugacy. The saccade from the patient with ocular myasthenia is initially conjugate (black arrow) but subsequently very disjunctive. The saccade from the patient with oculomotor nerve palsy is disjunctive from the onset (gray arrow). Eye movements were recorded using the magnetic search coil technique. Positive values on time plots indicate upward movements.

10 saccades and was then compared with the PI of the control subjects.

Representative records of an upward saccade from a control subject, a patient with ocular myasthenia, and a patient with oculomotor nerve palsy are shown in Figure 2. To the left in each row of the panels is a time plot; to the right are corresponding phase-plane plots of the upward saccades shown in the time plots. The vertical saccade made by the control subject (Fig. 2A) is tightly conjugate, as expected. The vertical saccade made by the patient with ocular myasthenia (Fig. 2B) is quite disjunctive, with greatly reduced movement of his left eye. However, as shown in the corresponding phase-plane plot, the upward saccade was initially conjugate (indicated by black arrow). In contrast, the saccade from the patient with oculomotor nerve palsy (Fig. 2C) was disjunctive throughout its course, including the onset (indicated by gray arrow on the phase-plane plot).

The three distinct patterns of vertical saccades were consistent from saccade to saccade when we systematically compared normalized phase planes of patients and control subjects: saccades of patients with ocular myasthenia invariably fell within the normal 95% prediction intervals for at least the first 10% of the movement (although later components did not), but saccades of patients with cranial nerve palsies always fell outside the normal 95% prediction intervals from their start. Similarly to what previously shown with horizontal saccades,[25] patients with ocular myasthenia exhibited a consistent initial interocular conjugacy of vertical saccades, from saccade to saccade, even though later components of saccades varied, reflecting fatigue.

Conclusions

Basic knowledge of physiological and pathological neuromuscular transmission can be applied to account for typical disorders of saccades encountered in ocular myasthenia. In health, the well-developed system of postsynaptic folding, which houses AChRs and NaChs, allows fidelity of neuromuscular transmission by determining an optimal magnitude of safety factor. Thus, the normal folding architecture of the postsynaptic membrane is instrumental in directing the current resulting from AChRs opening (at the crest of the primary folds) to an area of the membrane rich in NaChs (at the bottom of the secondary folds).[8] In myasthenia gravis,

the complement-mediated destruction of the postsynaptic membrane results in simplification of the folding system and depletion of AChRs and NaChs. This is ultimately responsible for the decrement of the endplate safety factor that translates in exercise-induced failure of neuromuscular transmission.[2,3] As opposed to regular skeletal muscle, the NMJ of five out of six categories of extraocular muscle fibers show physiologically poorly developed postsynaptic folding,[22] which would result in a lower baseline safety factor even in health. This could be an important factor to account for the common occurrence of abnormal eye movements in myasthenia.[24] However, one type of EOM fibers, the pale global singly innervated fibers, have better developed synaptic folding (Fig. 1) and their baseline safety factor may be higher than other EOM fiber types. The pale global fibers are believed to exert their function at the beginning of the eye movement, when their firing rate briefly increases, and are probably responsible for the initial high-acceleration component of saccades. The observation that the initial component of saccades remains binocularly conjugate in MG supports the hypothesis that the activity of the PGSF is relatively preserved in the disease due to their structural characteristics. Finally, the relative preserved functioning of the PGSF in myasthenia gravis might also account for the pathognomic clinical finding of "quiver movements," where eye movements are typically still fast despite having a markedly restricted range of motion.[29]

Acknowledgments

The Office of Research and Development, Medical Research Service, Department of Veterans Affairs (A.S., R.L.R., and R.J.L.); NIH Grant EY06717 and the Evenor Armington Fund (R.J.L.); Center of Excellence support from the Office of Rehabilitation Research of the Research and Development Service of the Department of Veterans Affairs (R.L.R.).

Conflicts of interests

The authors declare no conflicts of interest.

References

1. Soltys, J., B. Gong, H.J. Kaminski, *et al.* 2008. Extraocular muscle suceptibility to myasthenia gravis: unique immunological environment? *Ann. N.Y. Acad. Sci.* **1132:** 220–224.
2. Ruff, R.L. & V.A. Lennon. 2008. How myasthenia gravis alters the safety factor for neuromuscular transmission. *J. Neuroimmunol.* **15:** 201–202.

3. Serra, A., R. Ruff, H. Kaminski & R.J. Leigh. 2011. Factors contributing to failure of neuromuscular transmission in myasthenia gravis and the special case of the extraocular muscles. *Ann. N.Y. Acad. Sci.* **1233:** 26–33.

4. Angelides, K.J. 1986. Fluorescently labeled Na+ channels are localized and immobilized to synapses of innervated muscle fibers. *Nature* **321:** 63–66.

5. Flucher, B.E. & M.P. Daniels. 1989. Distribution of Na+ channels and ankyrin in neuromuscular junctions is complementary to that of acetylcholine receptors and the 43 kD protein. *Neuron* **3:** 163–175.

6. Haimovich, B., D.L. Schotland & R.L. Barchi. 1987. Localization of sodium channel subtypes in rat skeletal muscle using channel-specific monoclonal antibodies. *J. Neurosci.* **7:** 2957–2966.

7. Leteut, T., J.-L. Boudier, E. Jover & P. Cau. 2011. Localization of voltage-sensitive sodium channels on the extrasynaptic membrane surface of mouse skeletal muscle by autoradiography of scorpion toxin binding sites. *J. Neurocytol.* **19:** 408–420.

8. Slater, C.R. 2007. Structural factors influencing the efficacy of neuromuscular transmission. *Ann. N.Y. Acad. Sci.* **1132:** 1–12.

9. Engel, A.G. & G. Fumagalli. 1982. Mechanisms of acetylcholine receptor loss from the neuromuscular junction. *Ciba Found. Symp.* **90:** 197–224.

10. Engel, A.G., J.M. Lindstrom, E.H. Lambert & V.A. Lennon. 1977. Ultrastructural localization of the acetylcholine receptors in myasthenia gravis and in its experimental autoimmune model. *Neurology* **27:** 307–315.

11. Fambrough, D.M., D.B. Drachman & S. Satyamurti. 1973. Neuromuscular junction in myasthenia gravis: decreased acetylcholine receptors. *Science* **182:** 293–295.

12. Kaminski, H.J. & R.L. Ruff. 1999. Structure and kinetic properties of the acetylcholine receptor. In *Myasthenia Gravis and Myasthenic Syndromes.* A.G. Engel, Ed.: 40–64 Oxford University Press. New York.

13. Kao, I. & D. Drachman. 1977. Myasthenic immunoglobulin accelerates acetylcholine receptor degradation. *Science* **196:** 526–528.

14. Ruff, R.L. & V.A. Lennon. 1998. Endplate voltage-gated sodium channels are lost in clinical and experimental myasthenia gravis. *Ann. Neurol.* **43:** 370–279.

15. Engel, A.G. & T. Santa. 1971. Histometric analysis of the ultrastructure of the neuromuscular junction in myasthenia gravis and the myasthenic syndrome. *Ann. N.Y. Acad. Sci.* **183:** 46–63.

16. Santa, T., A.G. Engel & E.H. Lambert. 1972. Histometric study of neuromuscular junction ultrastructure: I. Myasthenia gravis. *Neurology* **22:** 71–82

17. Kaminski, H.J. & R.L. Ruff. 1996. The myasthenic syndromes. In *Physiology of Membrane Disorders.* S.G. Schultz, T.E. Andreoli, A.M. Brown, *et al.,* Eds.: 565–593. Plenum Press. New York.

18. Lennon, V.A. & E.H. Lambert. 1980. Myasthenia gravis induced by monoclonal antibodies to acetylcholine receptors. *Nature* **285:** 238–240.

19. Lindstrom, J.M., B.L. Einarson, V.A. Lennon & M.E. Seybold. 1976. Pathological mechanisms in experimental autoimmune myasthenia gravis: I. Immunogenicity of syngeneic muscle acetylcholine receptor and quantitative extraction of receptor and anti-receptor complexes from muscle of rats with experimental autoimmune myasthenia gravis. *J. Exp. Med.* **144:** 726–738.

20. Lindstrom, J.M., A.G. Engel, M.E. Seybold, *et al.* 1976. Pathological mechanisms in experimental autoimmune myasthenia gravis: II. Passive transfer of experimental autoimmune myasthenia gravis in rats with anti-acetylcholine receptor antibodies. *J. Exp. Med.* **144:** 739–753.

21. Maselli, R.A., D.P. Richman & R.L. Wollmann. 1991. Inflammation at the neuromuscular junction in myasthenia gravis. *Neurology* **41:** 1497–1504.

22. Spencer, R.F. & J.D. Porter. 2006. Biological organization of the extraocular muscles. *Prog. Brain. Res.* **151:** 33–79.

23. Scott, A.B. & C.C. Collins. 1973. Division of labor in human extraocular muscle. *Arch. Ophthalmol.* **90:** 319–322.

24. Khanna, S., K. Liao, H.J. Kaminski, *et al.* 2007. Myasthenia revisited: new insights from pseudo-internuclear ophthalmoplegia. *J. Neurol.* **254:** 1569–1574.

25. Serra, A., K. Liao, M. Matta & R.J. Leigh. 2008. Diagnosing disconjugate eye movements: phase-plane analysis of horizontal saccades. *Neurology* **71:** 1167–1175.

26. Leigh, R.J. & D.S. Zee. 2006. *The Neurology of Eye Movements, Book/DVD.* 4th ed. Oxford University Press. New York.

27. Moschovakis, A.K., C.A. Scudder & S.M. Highstein. 1990. A structural basis for Hering's law: projections to extrocular motoneurons. *Science* **248:** 1118–1119.

28. Ramat, S., J.T. Somers, V.E. Das & R.J. Leigh. 1999. Conjugate ocular oscillations during shifts of the direction and depth of visual fixation. *Invest. Ophthalmol. Vis. Sci.* **40:** 1681–1686.

29. Cogan, D.G., R.D. Yee & J. Gittinger. 1976. Rapid eye movements in myasthenia gravis: I. Clinical observations. *Arch. Ophthalmol.* **94:** 1083–1085.